FIRESIDE

Also by Gayle Olinekova
Go for It!
Legs!

To the hope that our seeking hearts will always find the true gentleness that comes from strength.

THE SENSUALITY OF STRENGTH
BY GAYLE OLINEKOVA

Photography Editor: MICHAEL GRANDI

A FIRESIDE BOOK
Published by Simon & Schuster, Inc.
New York

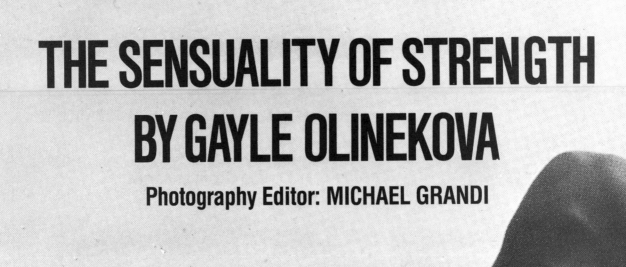

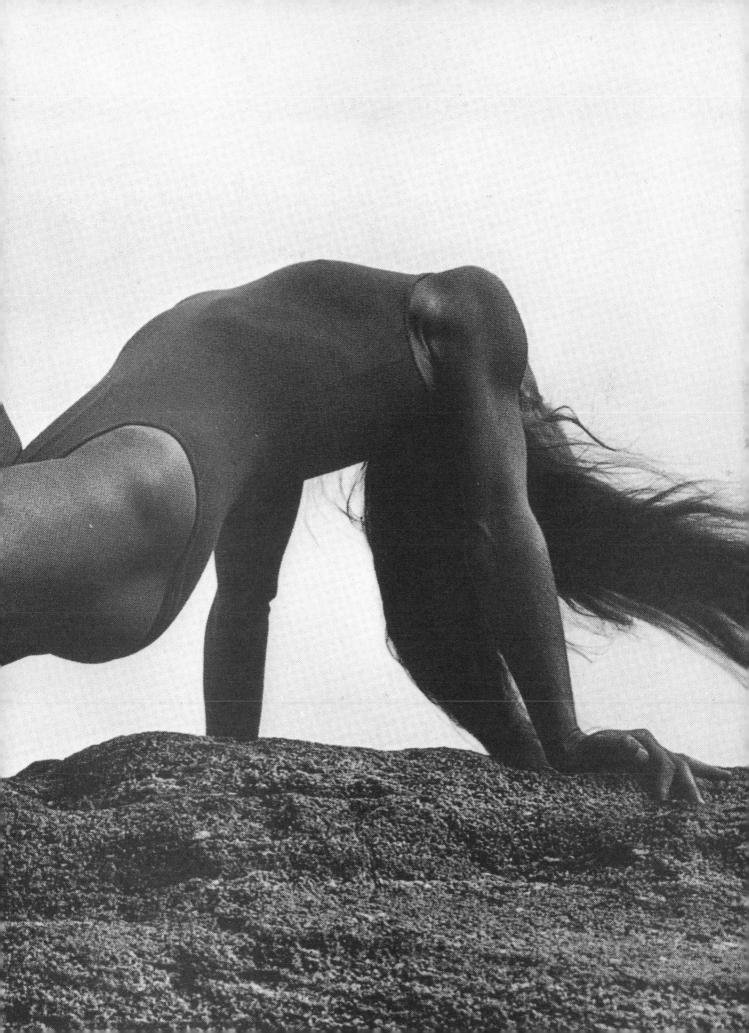

The instructions and advice in this book are in no way intended as a substitute for medical counseling. We advise anyone to consult with a doctor before beginning this or any other exercise regimen. The author and the publisher disclaim any liability or loss, personal or otherwise, resulting from the procedures in this book.

The author wishes to thank Roni's Gym, Florida, and The Buccaneer Hotel, St. Croix, for use of their facilities.

Equipment provided by Olinekova Fitness Centers, St. Croix and St. Thomas, U.S. Virgin Islands

Illustration: Exercise line drawings by Sabina Bronner-Lebovitz

Typing: Edith Butler

Photo Credits

Page 14—Warmup suit in Keyrolan® of Arnel® triacetate/Fortrel® polyester

Page 15—Warmup suits of Keyrolan of Arnel triacetate/Fortrel polyester

Page 16—Sweatshirt of Comfort Fiber and cotton

Page 22—Tops of Fortrel polyester

Page 25—Tank top trim and miniskirt in Super-Suede® of Arnel triacetate and nylon

Color Photo Credits

Cover—Alex Chatelaine (two-piece lounging pajamas in Ceylon® yarn of Fortrel® polyester)

Page 1—Alex Chatelaine (two-piece lounging pajamas in Ceylon yarn of Fortrel polyester)

Page 2—Alex Chatelaine (two-piece dress in Arnel triacetate/nylon)

Page 3, top—Alex Chatelaine (warmup suit in Action Suede® of Arnel® triacetate/Fortrel polyester)

Page 3, bottom—Alex Chatelaine (jacket and jeans of Fortrel ESP® stretch polyester/cotton)

Page 4—Michael Grandi (sweatshirts of Comfort Fiber/cotton)

Page 5—Alex Chatelaine (warmup suit in Keyrolan® of Arnel triacetate/Fortrel polyester)

Page 6, top—Alex Chatelaine (Arnel triacetate robe)

Page 6, bottom—Alex Chatelaine (evening dress in Arnel triacetate/nylon)

Page 7, top—Alex Chatelaine (sweatshirt of Comfort Fiber/cotton and jeans of Fortrel ESP stretch polyester/cotton)

Page 7, bottom—Michael Grandi (stretch leotard of Fortrel polyester/cotton)

Page 8, top left—Alex Chatelaine (jacket in Polarfleece™ of Fortrel polyester and jeans of Fortrel ESP stretch polyester/cotton)

Page 8, top right—Alex Chatelaine (shirt of Comfort Fiber/cotton and jeans of Fortrel ESP stretch polyester/cotton)

Page 8, bottom—Alex Chatelaine (warmup suit in Action Suede of Arnel triacetate/Fortrel polyester)

Back Cover—Michael Grandi

Black-and-White Photo Credits

Alex Chatelaine: pages 14, 15, 16, 22, 23, 25

Michael Grandi: pages 4–5, 12, 13, 18, 19, 20, 21, 28, 30, 32, 33, 34, 36, 37, 38, 39, 40, 41, 42, 43, 44, 45, 46, 48, 49, 50, 51, 52, 53, 54, 55, 56, 57, 60, 64, 65, 66, 67, 68, 88, 91, 92, 93, 94, 98, 102, 103, 111

Don Lauritzen: pages 26, 28, 29

Richard Mackson: pages 58–59

Contents

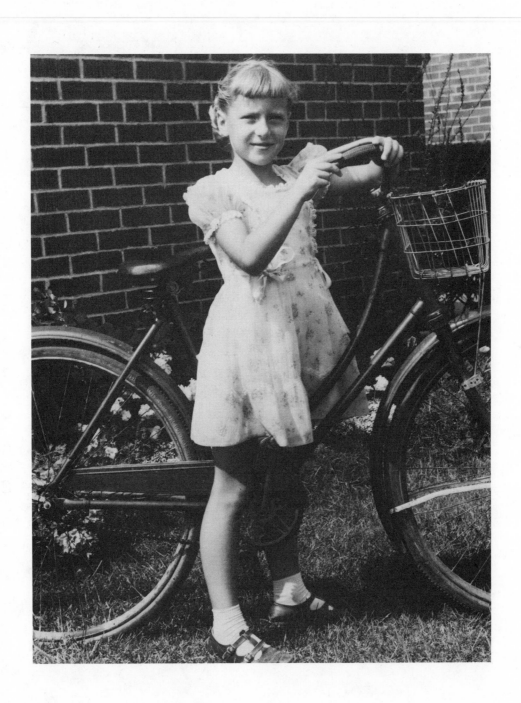

Introduction

This book is about you. You are here today because two people cared enough about each other to merge their very cells together. Of the millions of choices available, you were created.

You are special and unique. Your body is more than just the place where you live. It is a vehicle for expressing all of your emotions and sensations. It knows limitless possibilities, from the touch of love to the fist of pain. Our bodies can transmit an abundance of continually renewable pleasures—if we allow them to.

Yet do you allow yourself all the pleasures your body can give? Are you holding out on yourself—too tired to cope, shuffling through life without ever feeling the power and energy of being totally fit? You don't have to be an Olympic athlete to have the A-1, top-of-the-line model when it comes to your body.

This book is for you. In it, I will share many of the feelings I've come to know living inside an athletic body. Even if you can only give yourself twenty minutes a day, the same feelings can be yours. If you're already following an exercise program, keep up the good work. But if you've yet to start, keep turning pages. Become a new you, starting today.

Your once in a lifetime is right now. Someday you'll have the body you've always wanted. A body with every possible convenience and luxury—built to your exact specifications.

Just once in your life, let it be now.

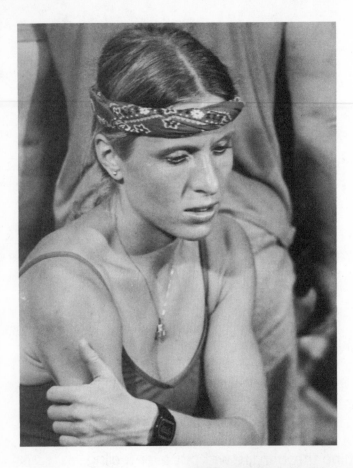

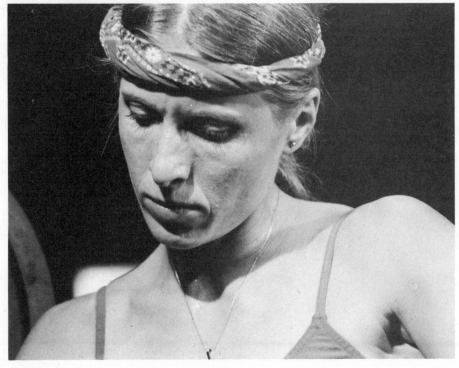

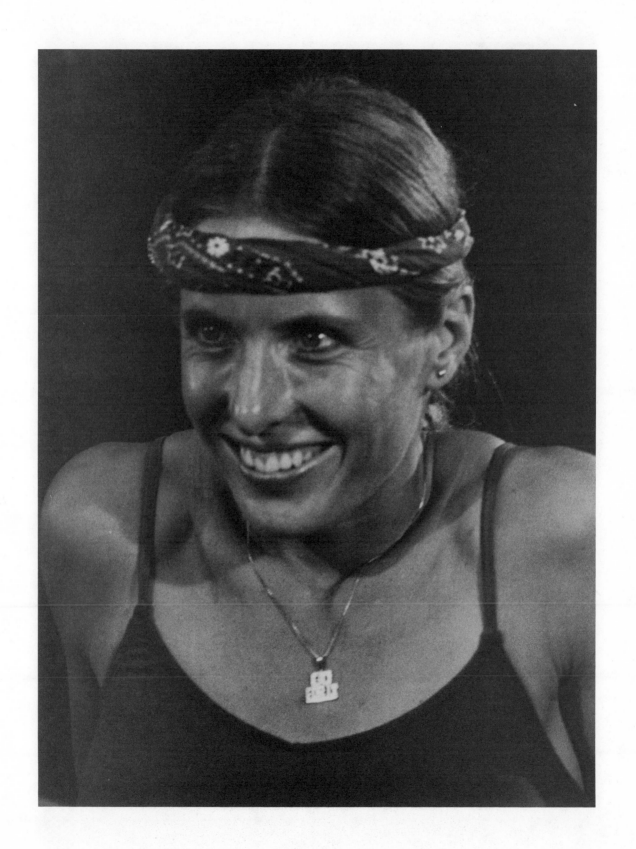

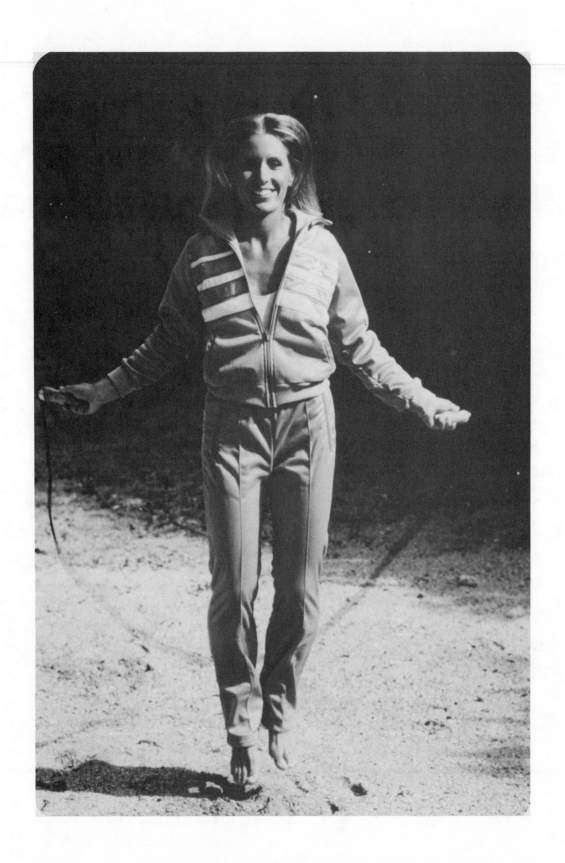

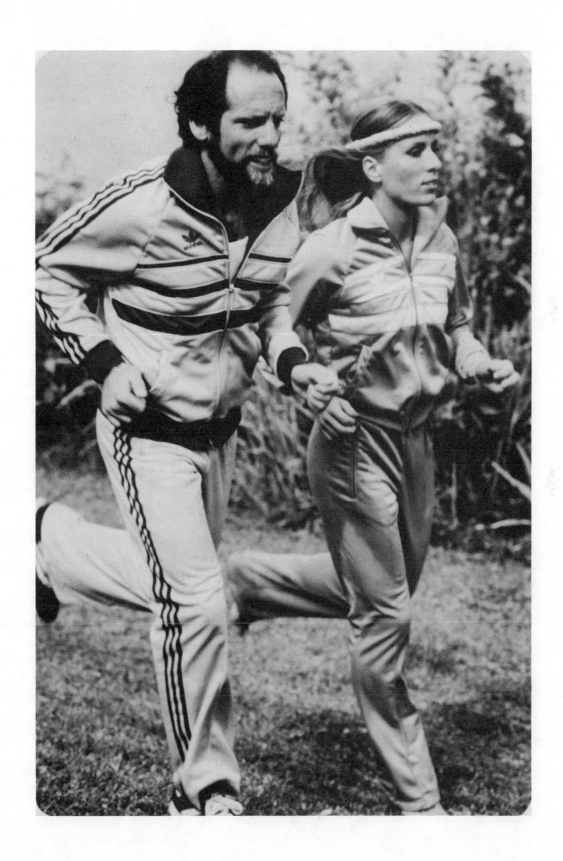

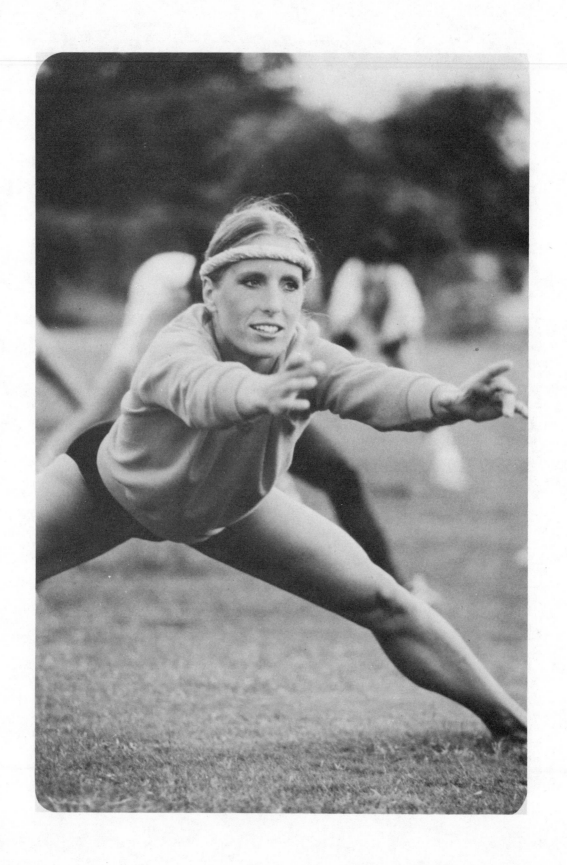

Steps to an Athletic Body Beautiful

Set a goal for yourself and then go for it. (Need I say more?)

Be realistic. Rome wasn't built in one week, and that goes for you, too. So start more than a week before your high school reunion.

Make better choices for yourself. You have free will —use it.

Live in the present. Let go of the past—you don't need it any longer. Be **here** today. Wake up in the morning ready to give fresh thoughts air time instead of old scenarios.

Listen to your instincts. On your first day at the ski slope, you don't have to schuss down Devil's Peak just because everyone else is doing it.

Similarly, if you're having trouble shuffling to the bathroom first thing in the morning because you over-did it in yesterday's aerobic class, listen to your body. Take it easy today. Perhaps a few laps in the pool would do the trick for you instead. But listen to your body.

Do something creative every day. It's simple. No matter how small a creative activity it is, it has the power to obliterate destructive tendencies. Whether it's making up a new bedtime story for your kids, planting a few marigolds, or painting a cathedral wall—do it.

Forgive yourself. You say you gave yourself an Iroquois punk hairstyle and then dyed it green on St. Patrick's Day? And now you hate it? At least you know what style **not** to get in the future.

Forgive yourself your past mistakes, and give yourself permission to try, try again.

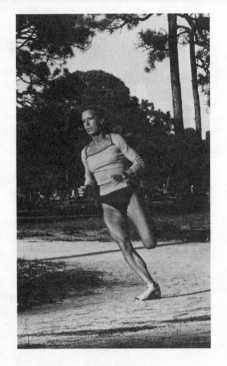

License to succeed. To drive a car, you need a license. The same goes for succeeding. You must give yourself **permission** to achieve that athletic body beautiful. The possibilities are dazzling.

But just as you don't wheel into the Indy 500 your first day behind the wheel, don't expect to be ready to win the Olympic final your first day, either.

Take pleasure in **getting there**, not just in the results. Give yourself permission to enjoy each small triumph—your first chin-up, even your first attempt at a sit-up.

Stand tall and be a winner. Posture, posture, **posture!** Have you ever seen royalty slouch or sag? You are like royalty—treat yourself with that kind of respect. Hold your head high. Check yourself out during the day. Be conscious of what your body language is saying about you. Make it say how proud and worthy a person you are.

Go for it. Undoubtedly, we could make excuses for **not** doing just about anything. But there comes a time when you have to just suck it in and **do it anyway**. The big surprise will be that not only **can** you do it, but you **are** doing it, and you're **good** at it!

Keep laughing. For one thing, laughing really develops the abdominal muscles—something I can personally attest to.

In addition, laughing with, and even at, yourself keeps you from becoming a crashing bore to your friends and colleagues. I was once told that possibly the worst criticism of any human had to be "She/He has absolutely no sense of humor."

Life becomes bitter without laughter, and as the **Reader's Digest** column maintains, "Laughter is the best medicine." In fact, Norman Cousins, famed editor-in-chief of the **Saturday Review**, actually cured himself of cancer by a whole program of feeling better for himself which started with watching reruns of funny movies all day.

Have some fun getting there, and **do** try to get in a few laughs every day.

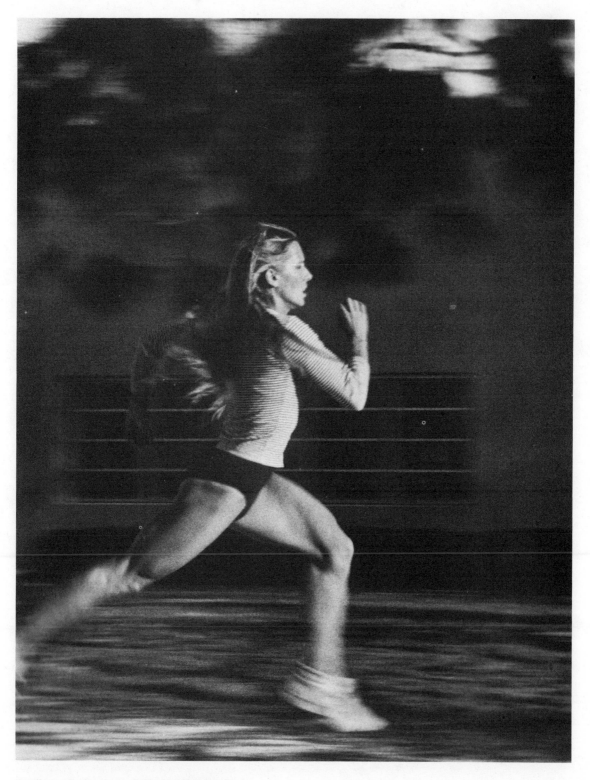

Feeling my body quietly tuning itself

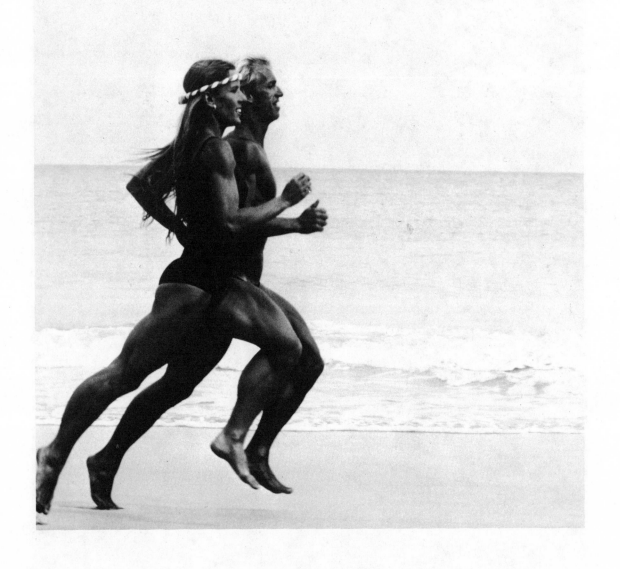

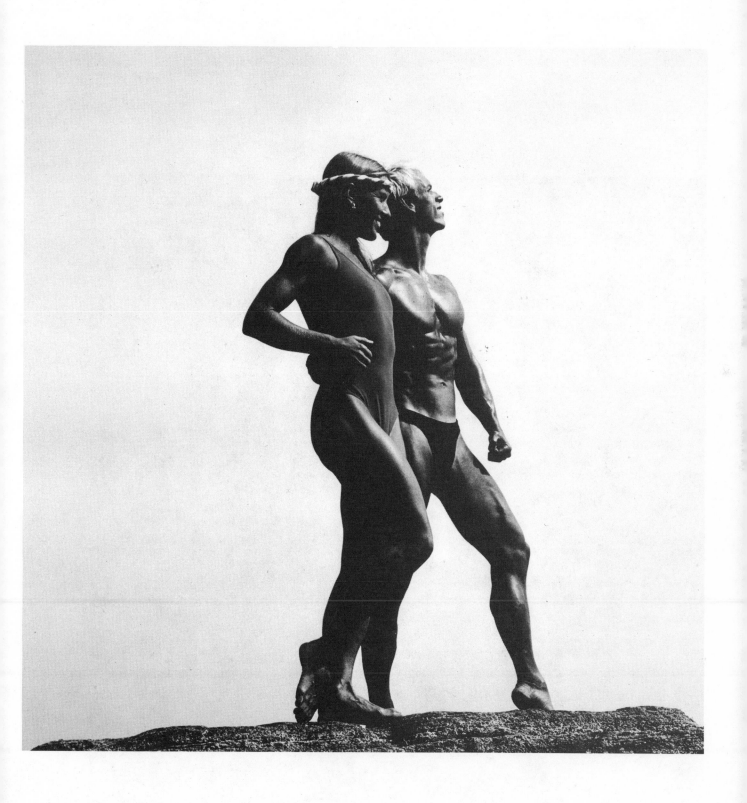

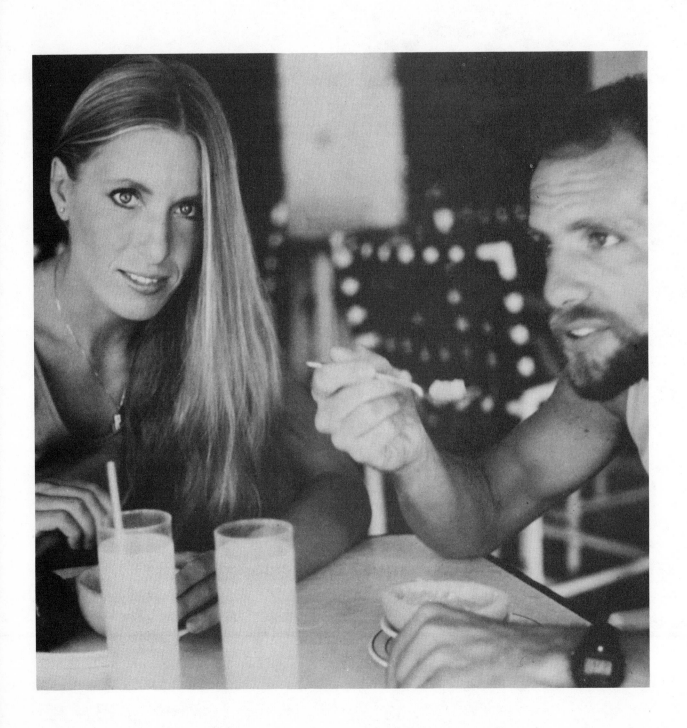

Food

Eat only when you are hungry enough to be grateful for your food. If you're not that hungry, don't eat.

The French expression **bon appétit** is said in many languages before a meal. It's a good expression because what it really means is "may you eat with a good appetite."

After all is said about food preparation and planning, the fact is that if you're not **really** hungry, nothing tastes good. But even the simplest piece of fruit can taste like nectar from the gods if you're truly in need of it.

And while we're on the topic of needs, let's discuss some of the needs that we all try to fill with food at some time or other.

Boredom, frustration, and depression are probably at the top of the list as causes of binge eating. We sometimes use food to try to fill the void that can exist in other parts of our lives. This happens when our minds and bodies are not coordinated and therefore work against each other.

Think of being in love. The high-flying happiness leaves no room for destructive binge eating, because at that time you are tuned in to the universal energy that has made the world turn for thousands of years. You sing in the shower. You smile at yourself in the mirror when you're brushing your teeth. You're in love.

Yet we all know the sometimes tenuous quality of love affairs. And if the phone doesn't ring, out comes the spoon and the half gallon of ice cream.

It doesn't have to be that way. You can depend upon **yourself** for that "love affair" energy. Start a lifetime relationship with **yourself** today. Work that body. Sweat. Use those muscles. And then come home hungry and eat good food with a good appetite. Guilt-free.

You'll soon find that you're making better choices for yourself in the food department as well as in all the other departments in your life. Better choices born of the self-respect and confidence that comes from loving yourself enough to take care of yourself.

The earth provides food for us. The trees lay their fruit down on the ground for us as a gift of life. And it behooves us to accept it, as any gift, with grateful hearts. The molecules of that food will become part of your body. So choose it with care and thanksgiving.

Superstar Thin Tips

- Eat only when you are hungry.
- Boredom is a main cause of overeating.
- Focus on non-food activities to release anger or depression—sex, for instance. It even burns calories.
- What you don't keep in the house you won't eat.
- Don't skip meals—you'll only get grouchy and end up over-compensating at the next meal.
- Make better choices for yourself—you know what they are.
- Don't ever expect to "oink out."
- If you've got it, you might just as well flaunt it—stand up straight—pull in your stomach.
- Act as though you're already thin.
- Eat slowly.
- Don't eat while you're watching TV or reading. Eating itself should be entertainment enough.

Sensuality of Strength

- Firmer confidence (but not cockiness) makes one more attractive to others.
- A body that is attractive and in good condition is a turn-on to others. Physically one is a better lover for it.
- A well-conditioned body responds with greater sensitivity to all aspects of life, air, sleep, food and the small pleasures of being alive—and with greater sensuality to others.
- Your positive energy will reflect and turn on others. It will turn on the person in you as you tap the power of sensuality within.

Happiness in the form of sustained work on your own body—physical
work that leads to self respect and eating with care.

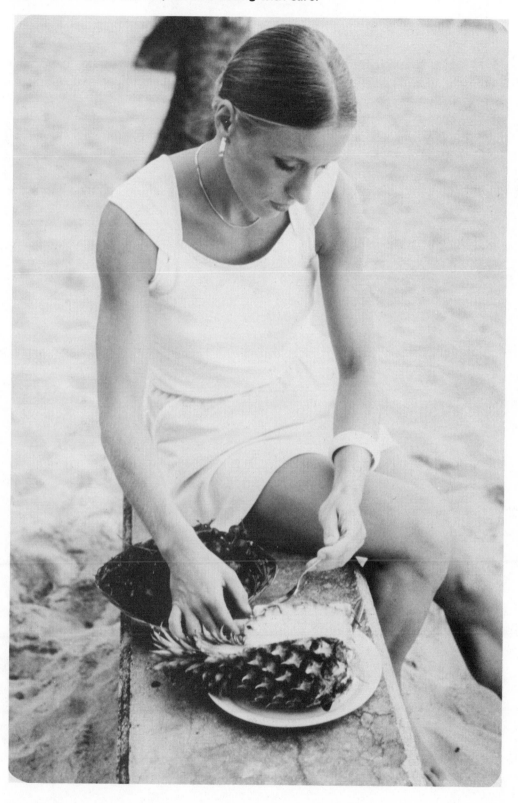

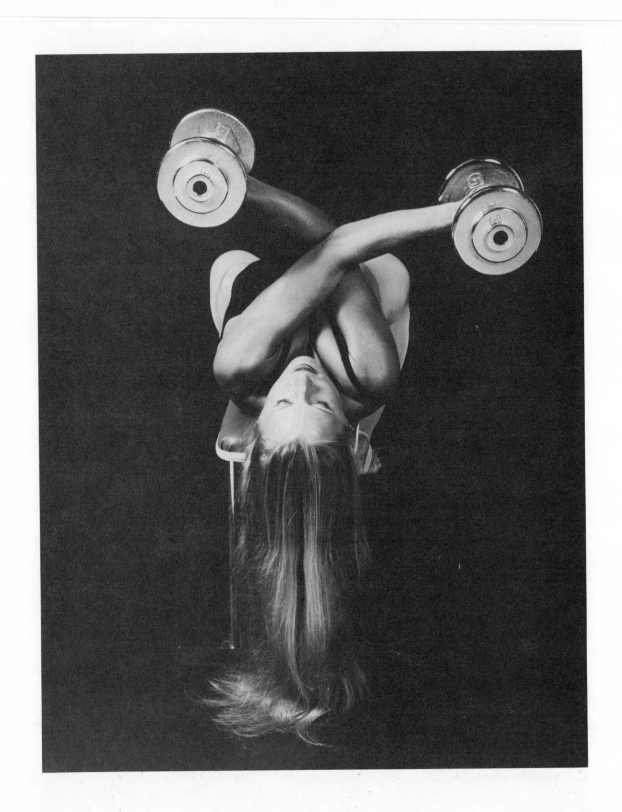

Sex

Before you ever know a person's name, and long after you've forgotten it, you'll still remember the first observation of that person—whether male or female.

In our culture we often define sexuality in the narrow sense—the frame of reference restricted to genital stimulation and reproductive motives.

But sex is not just something a person does. It extends far beyond our cultural limitations of morality, machismo, and marriage.

Our hearts beat every moment. Our circulatory system works for us whether we think of it or not. Similarly, our sexual rhythms are in existence every moment, whether we choose to think of them or not.

Yet in our civilization we are taught to ignore our sexual energy whenever possible, although this is a contradiction of the life energy itself.

For instance, in our culture women cover their breasts. Yet the underwear worn—a bra—actually accentuates the form of the breast.

Clearly, our messages are confused. One code of behavior attempts to extinguish the sexual effect, and the other code ignites the denied effect.

Even the way we walk in North America—with frozen pelvis—says a lot about us. Conversely, in Mediterranean countries people walk swaying their hips, actually using the gluteus muscles of the derriere to fulfill the kinesiological function of the walking movement.

Movement itself is evocative. And more movement is even more evocative, simply because when we move we are forced to breathe deeply—to expand our bodies and be aware of their action.

Before a baby is even out of the womb, it kicks. Movement is our instinct—the beauty of it, the line of it, the physicality of it. There is our freedom.

To feel, we must breathe. What do we do when we

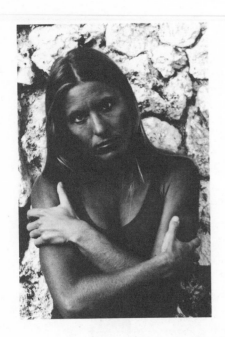

don't want to feel too much? We breathe shallow, lifeless little breaths.

How does all this relate to our sexuality? Sexual energy is like any other vehicle; it can take you anywhere—you're the driver.

Some people never take it past the bedroom. That's okay. But sexual energy is only generated from our reproductive organs. It is not confined there—it only originates there.

Our sexuality is expressed in so many other ways. We can experience it in every cell and pore of our body. Scientifically, our genetic inheritance, including the chromosomes—the male or female genetic blueprint— is actually **carried** by every cell in our bodies.

Sexuality is the creative, explorative life force. People have often tried to define masculinity or femininity in words, or in codes of behavior, but we are past the point where blue is just for little boys and pink is just for little girls.

Our sexual energy is a way of being, not only a way of doing. Music, dance, movement, sweat, heartbeats— these are all an extension of our sexual energy, just as a song, a scent, a poem, or a sculpture can also awaken and focus us with our life energy.

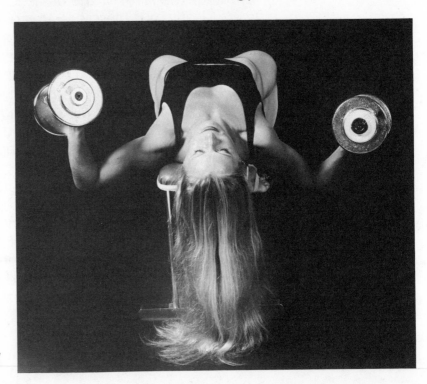

The image of a woman as a doll or decoration has finally given way to that of a woman exhilarated by her own strength.

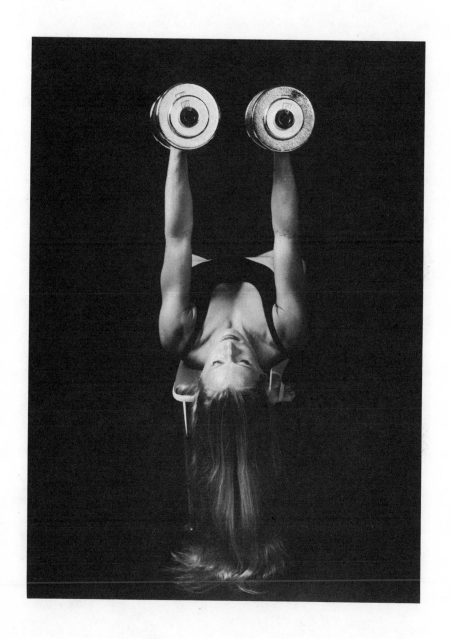

Let yourself move with the rhythms of life—not just in the bedroom, but with your own heartbeat. Exercise yourself. Move. Breathe deeply and inhale the energy of the universe—the healing heartbeat of life itself which can lift our spirits, our sexuality, our souls, into the world of the creative.

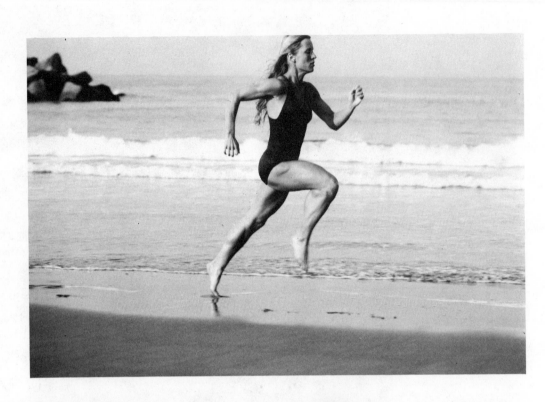

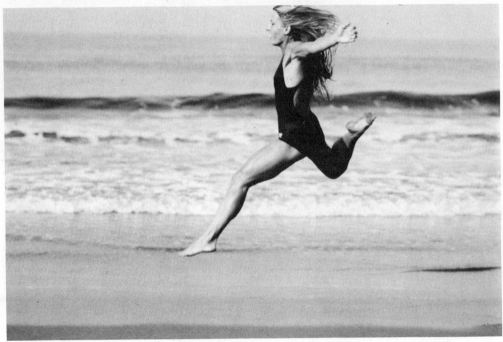

Breathing

Breathing is our most important physical function. If you don't believe it, try to stop it! The average person could survive more than thirty days without food, more than a week without water, but less than three minutes without breathing.

The air we breathe contains all the building blocks of the universe: air, light, fluids, and solids. We are actually breathing machines from the top of our heads to the soles of our feet—we breathe in and out from every pore.

Actually, breathing not only rids the lungs of wastes and poisons that cannot be thrown off any other way; the glands and organs themselves use breathing for this purpose, too. Breathing is the regulator that controls the metabolism.

And if breathing controls us physiologically, how far does it go in affecting us psychologically? Our brains require 20 percent of all the oxygen our bodies absorb through breathing in order to function. Thus, something as simple as the inflow and outflow of air into our lungs has the power to revitalize every cell in our bodies. And the shortcut to progress in any direction—whether it be health, greater achievement, or the ability to make decisions more successfully—lies in using our breath of life to the fullest.

Naturally, one of the definitions of fitness is the ability to process oxygen with maximum efficiency. That in itself slows down the aging process.

Here's a technique that will also allow you to increase your breathing powers. Either sit cross-legged or lie down. Loosen any tight clothing—especially around the waistline.

Take a breath very slowly, and when you think you have filled your lungs, squeeze more in. This strengthens your inhalation muscles.

Running barefoot on a beach, with the heady mix of warm sand and the salty sensuality of the ocean—here I find the rhythms, the very heartbeat of life.

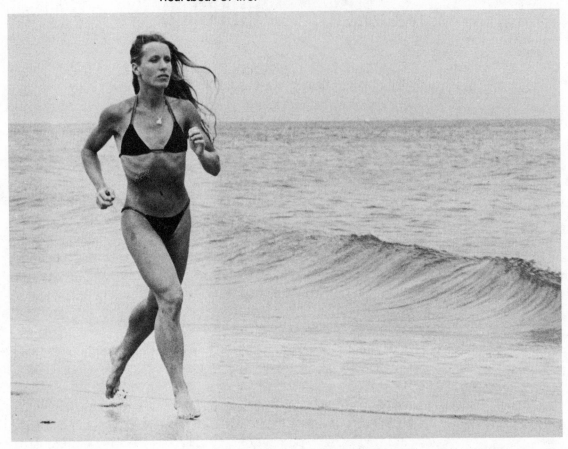

Then exhale slowly, and when you think you have gotten all the air out, force more out. This strengthens the muscles of exhalation.

Do all of the breathing **in** through your nose. Breathe out through your mouth.

Just take a few deep breaths like this at first. Then do it while you are walking, or at any other time you think of it.

Taking in air is the life force.

When you are born, you take the first breath; when you die, you give it back. But in between, use your breathing to the fullest. It is God-given, for the breath **is** life.

32

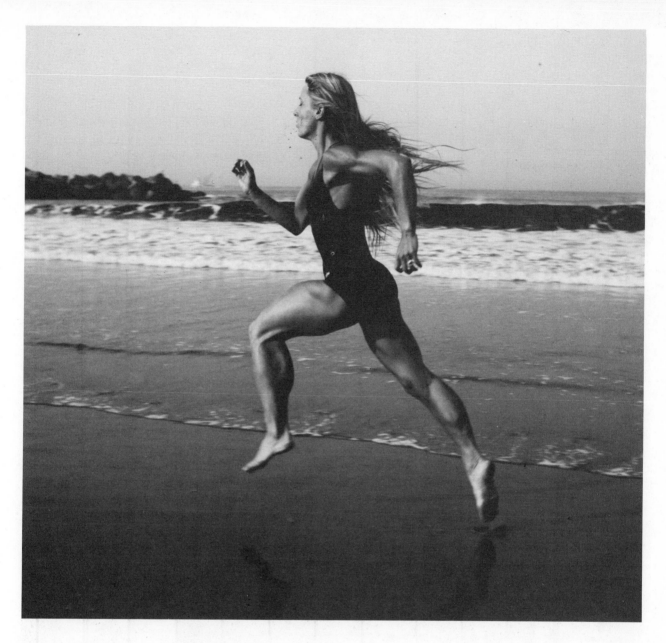

Breathing

Never hold your breath when lifting weights or doing an exercise.

Remember
> exhale during the exertion phase

> inhale during the return to the start position

EXAMPLE—Sit-ups
- Take in a deep breath when you're ready to start
- Breathe *out* when bringing the trunk toward the knees
- Breathe *in* when returning to start position

33

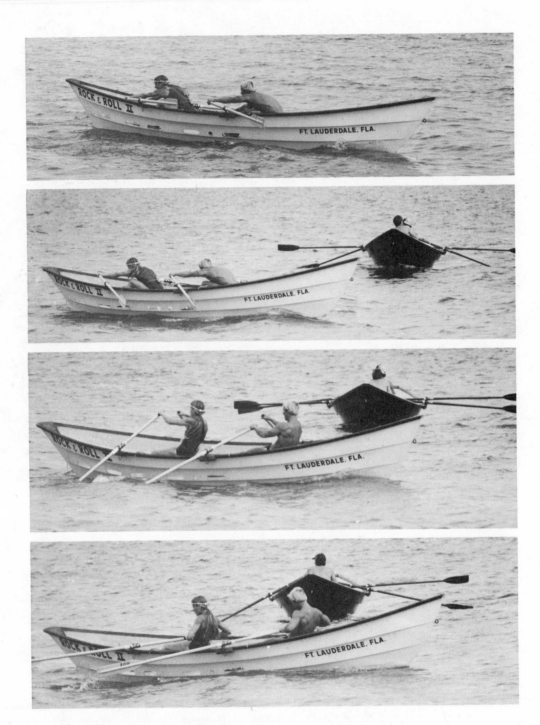

Rowing in the South Atlantic with Chuck Niessen, world-record holder in two ocean-rowing events

Sleep

Sleep "knits up the ravell'd sleave of care," Shakespeare wrote. It is also our time to revitalize the life energy. Our time to travel in the netherworlds of our subconscious and dream the Technicolor fantasies of a mind freed from the moment-to-moment tasks of daily caretaking.

Oriental philosophies embrace the idea that the vital force of the universe is received by our minds and bodies during sleep. Instant get-to-sleep therapy is just another great by-product of a body and mind coordinated.

One technique for slipping into slumberland is the following:

Lie flat on your back with a pillow under your knees. Practice a few deep breaths as outlined in the breathing section on page 00.

Now relax all of the muscles in your body one by one. Starting with your head and moving down— face, neck, shoulders, arms, chest, abdomen, fingertips, back, buttocks, legs, knees, feet, toes.

Be conscious of each body part becoming very heavy. Continue calm, relaxed breathing and feel your entire body slipping peacefully into quiet, restful calm.

If for some reason you cannot sleep, don't worry about it. Get up and use the time constructively. A warm bath is often helpful. Reading, stretching, or simple tidying up are other activities that can help. But **do** beware of "tidying up" the refrigerator. This is **not** a license to binge.

Think calm, beautiful thoughts at bedtime. Count your blessings, relax, and sweet dreams. . . .

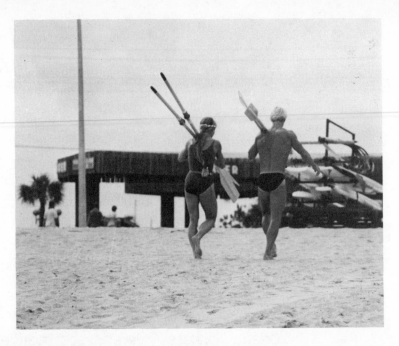

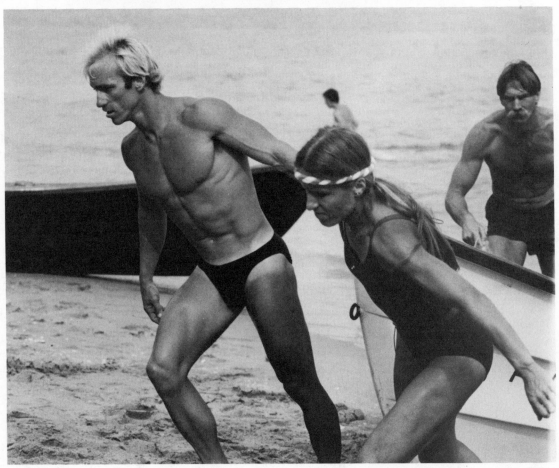

Triumph is just a try with a little "umph."

On Sleeping and Eating—A Few Tips

- Don't eat late at night before sleep.
- Don't eat a big meal when you're really tired.
- Sleep is as important as the training. Catch afternoon naps whenever possible. Even if you don't sleep, twenty minutes of complete relaxation lying down will refresh you for the evening workout. Ironically, the more you train, the more fitfully you sometimes sleep at night. The body is too exhausted to sleep. Listen to your body—it always tries to do the best thing for you. Naps help prevent the cycle of fatigue, which destroys your body, tearing down rather than building.

So take care of yourself.

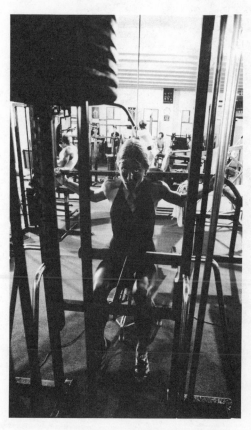

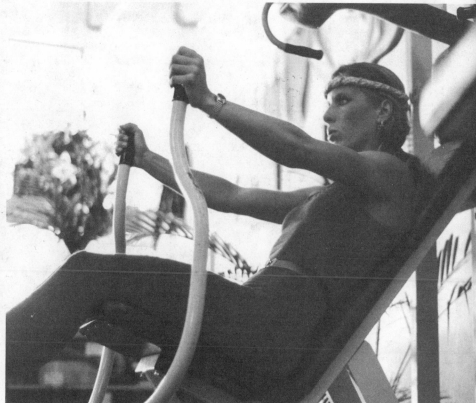

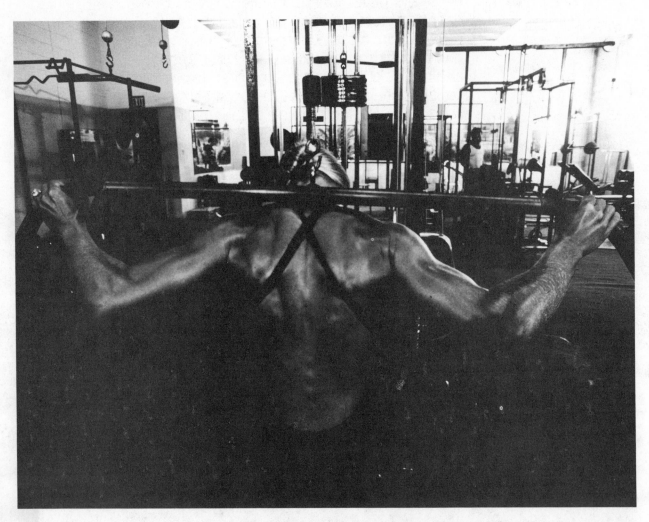

More than just a gym—an opportunity for technical refinement and the expression of strength with heavy metal

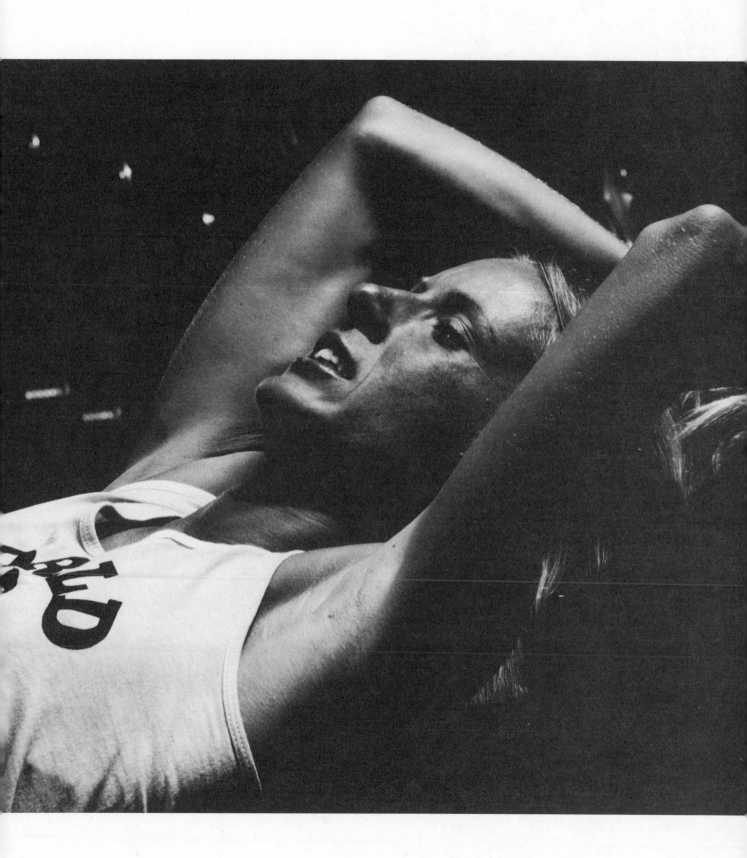

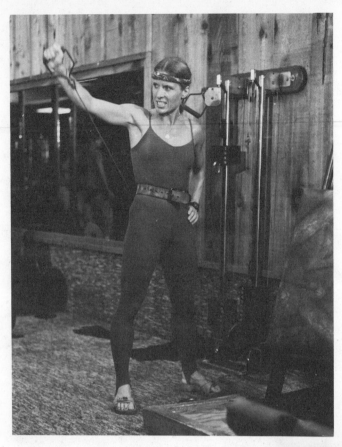

Why exercise? Because each of us
has a heart that yearns for the
immense and nourishing idea
of personal freedom.

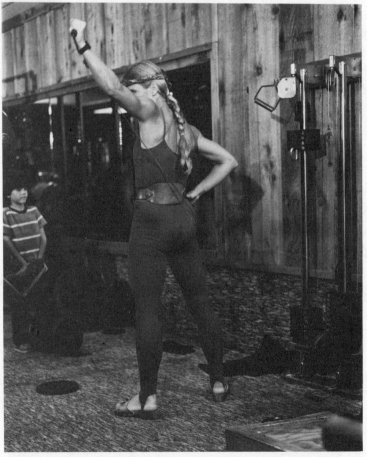

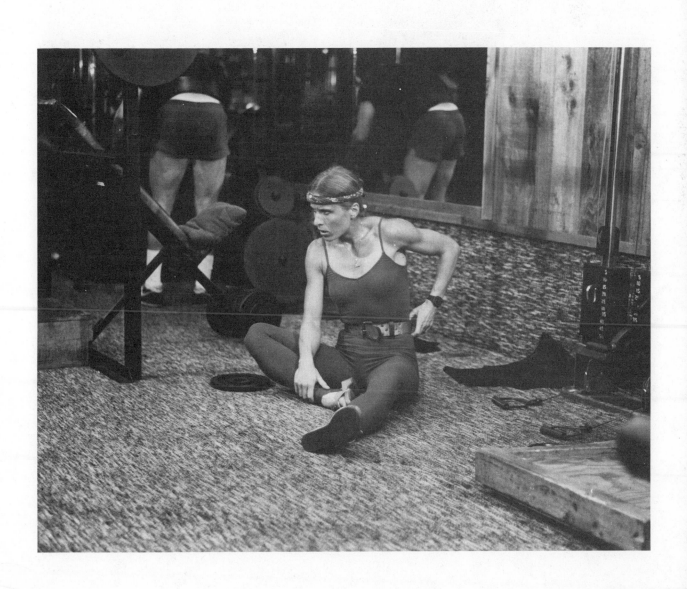

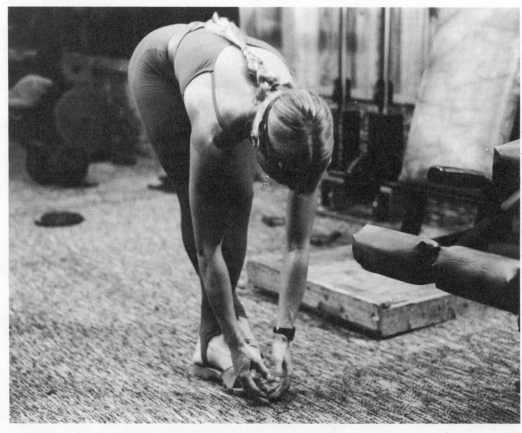
Getting stronger is mentally releasing your weaknesses and physically filling your body with strength and energy.

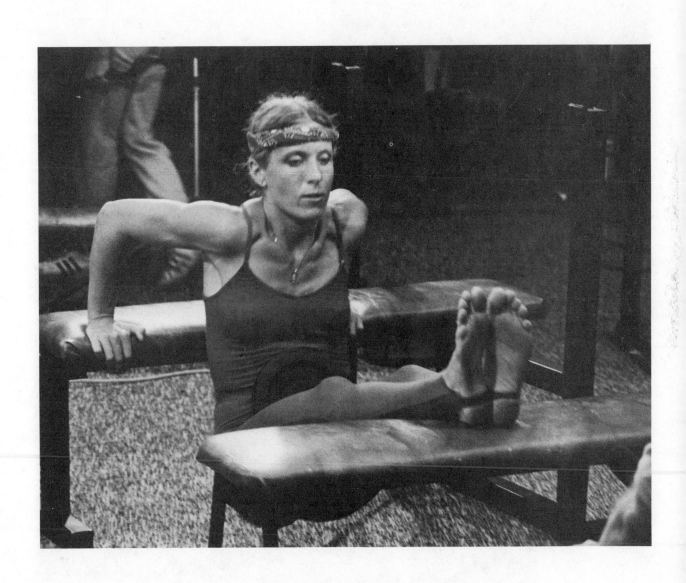

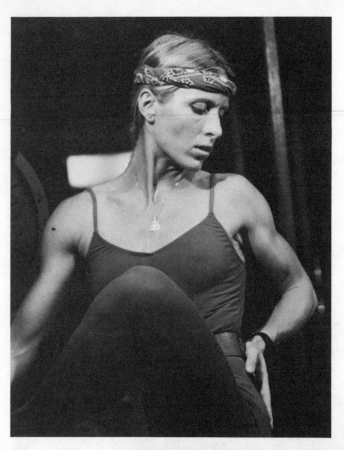

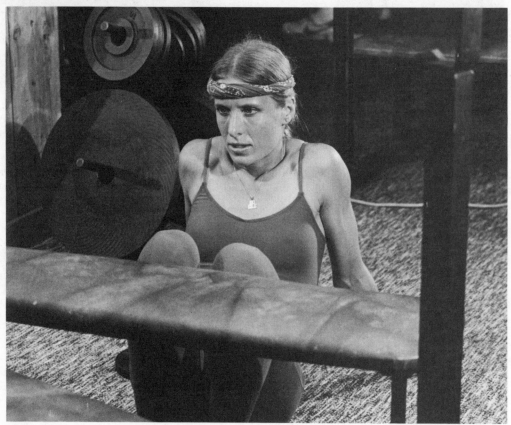

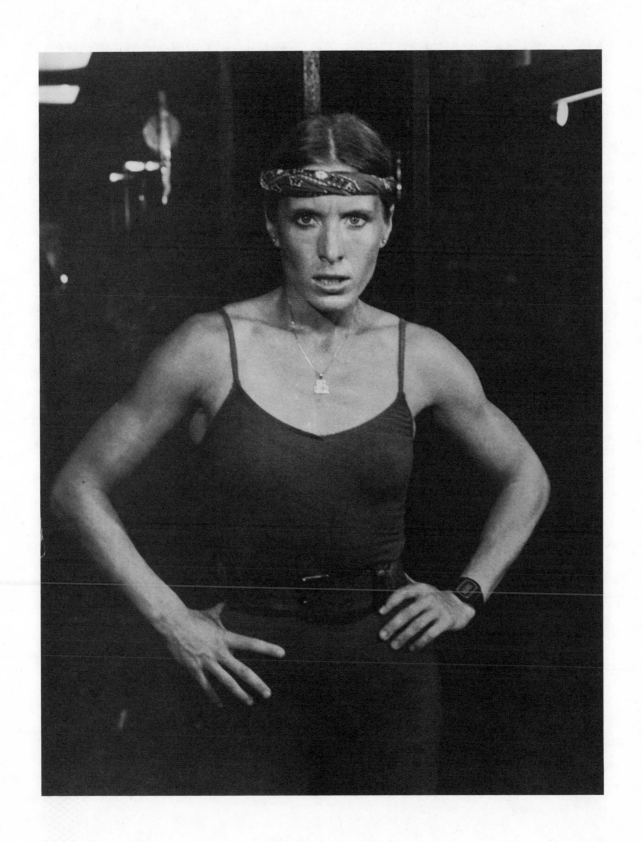

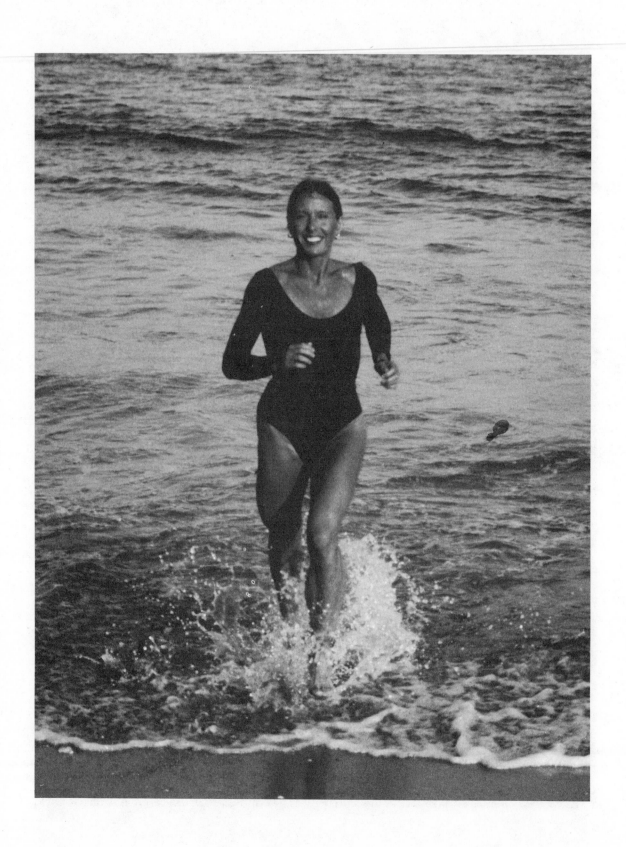

Fifteen Ways to Feel Great

1. Go for a long walk.

2. Sing to yourself in the shower today.

3. Relive your proudest moment.

4. Give away some of your old clothes to charity.

5. List all the stuff you like about yourself on paper.

6. Put on some terrific music and dance. Really get into it.

7. Tell someone you love her/him.

8. Take a bubble bath.

9. Forgive yourself for one of your past mistakes.

10. Forgive somebody else.

11. Count your blessings.

12. Send your favorite person a Christmas card—even if it's July.

13. Cut an obvious piece of junk food out of your diet.

14. Take a cold shower and let out a few Tarzan yells.

15. Decide to really get into shape—and then go for it!

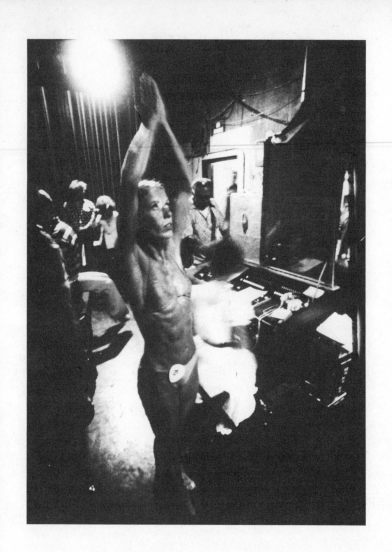

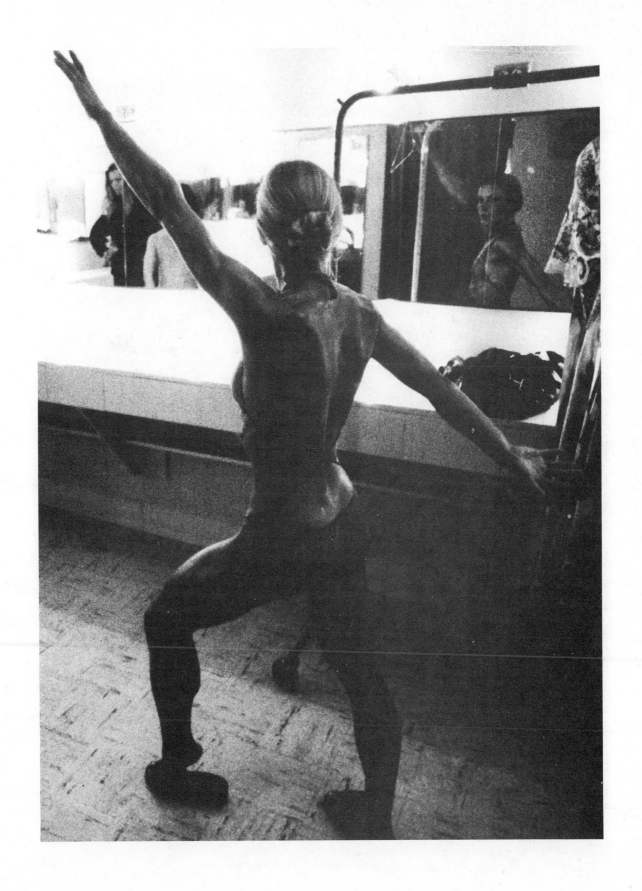

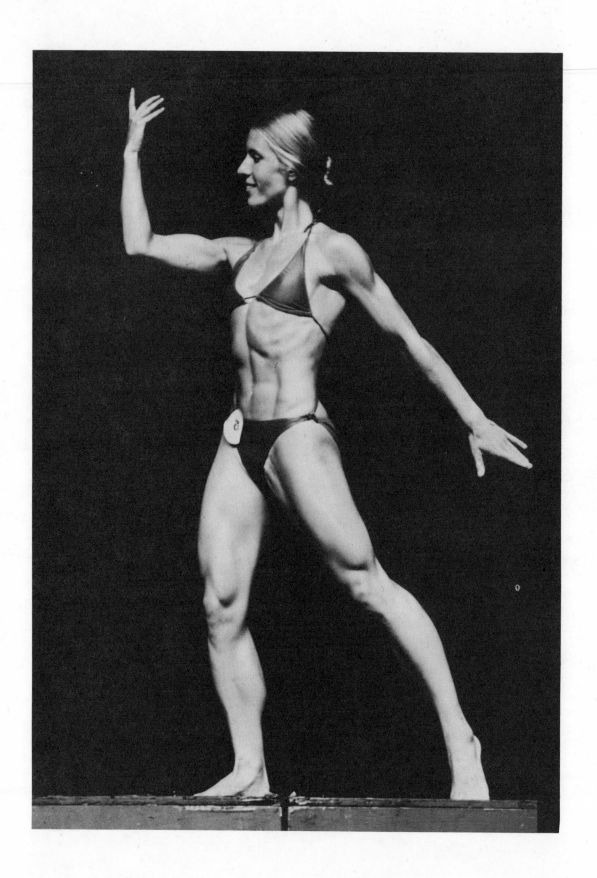

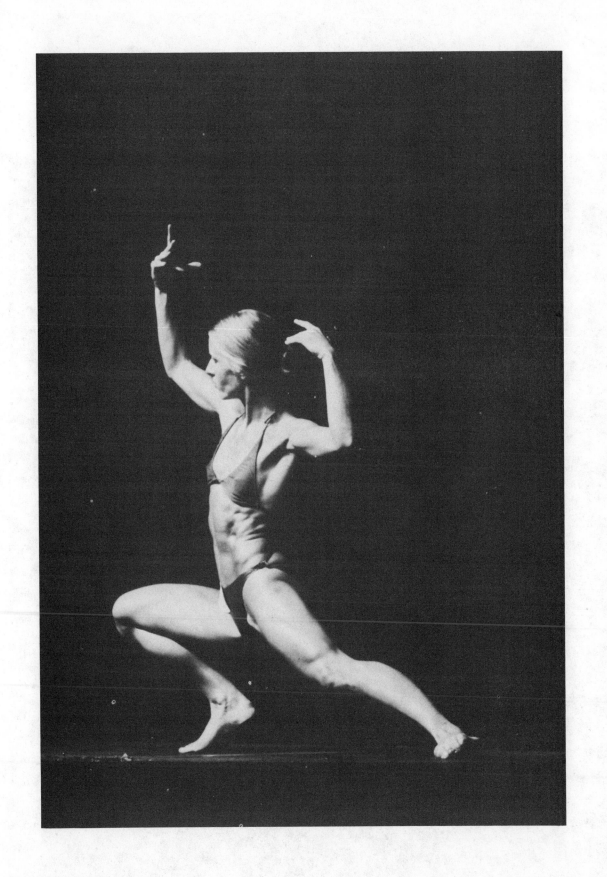

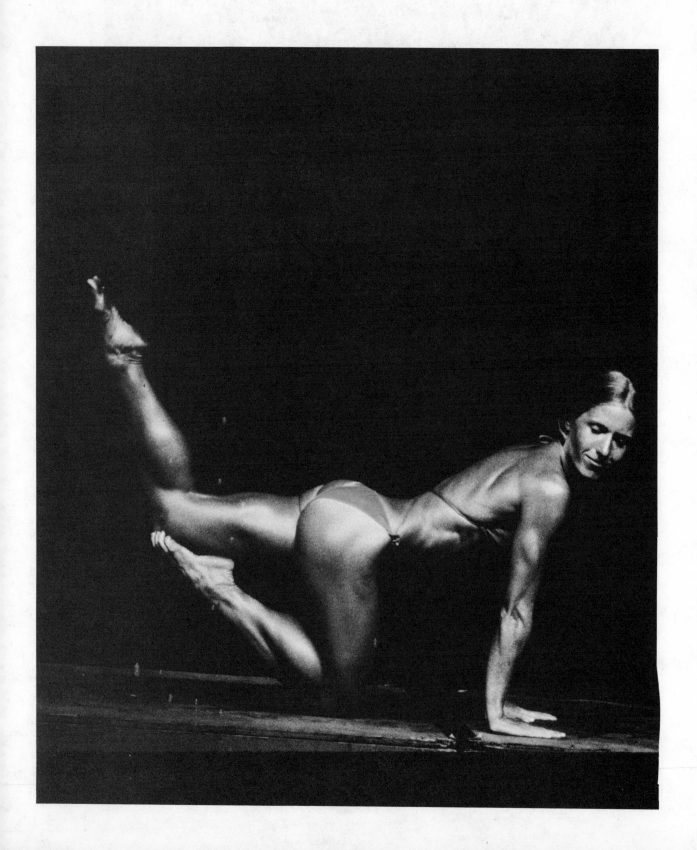

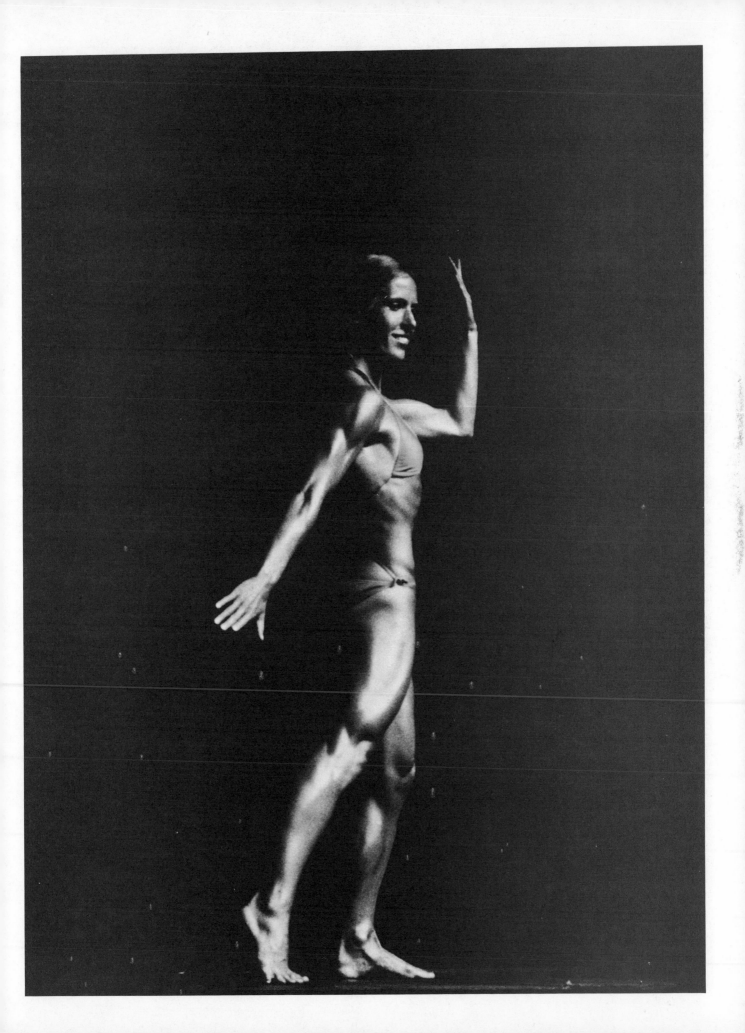

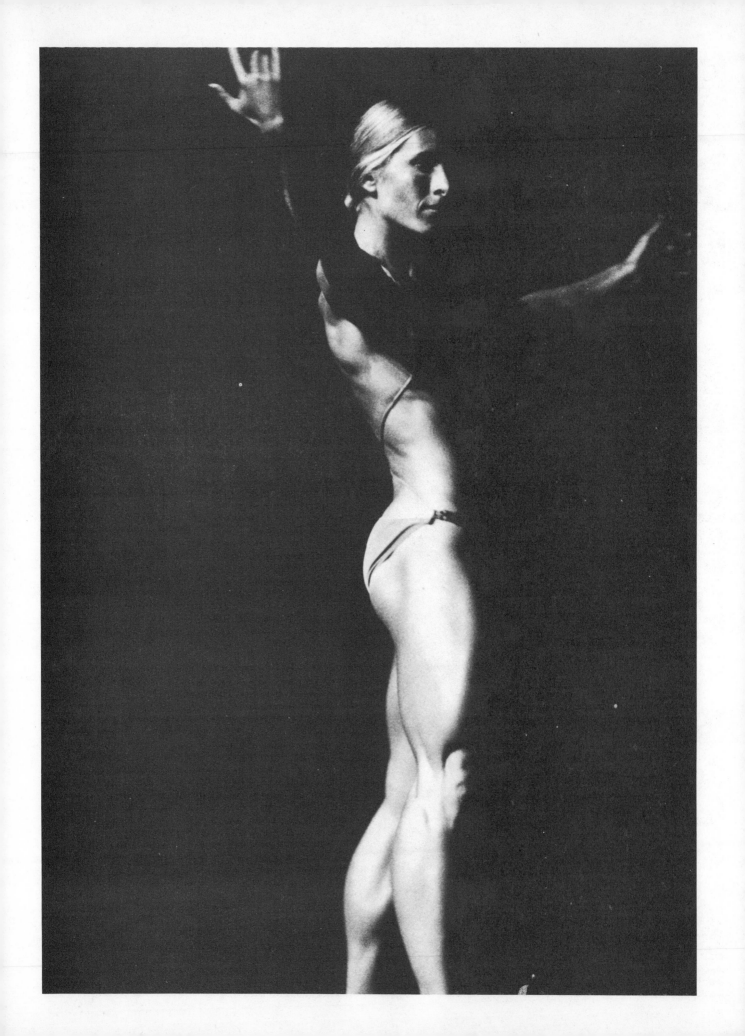

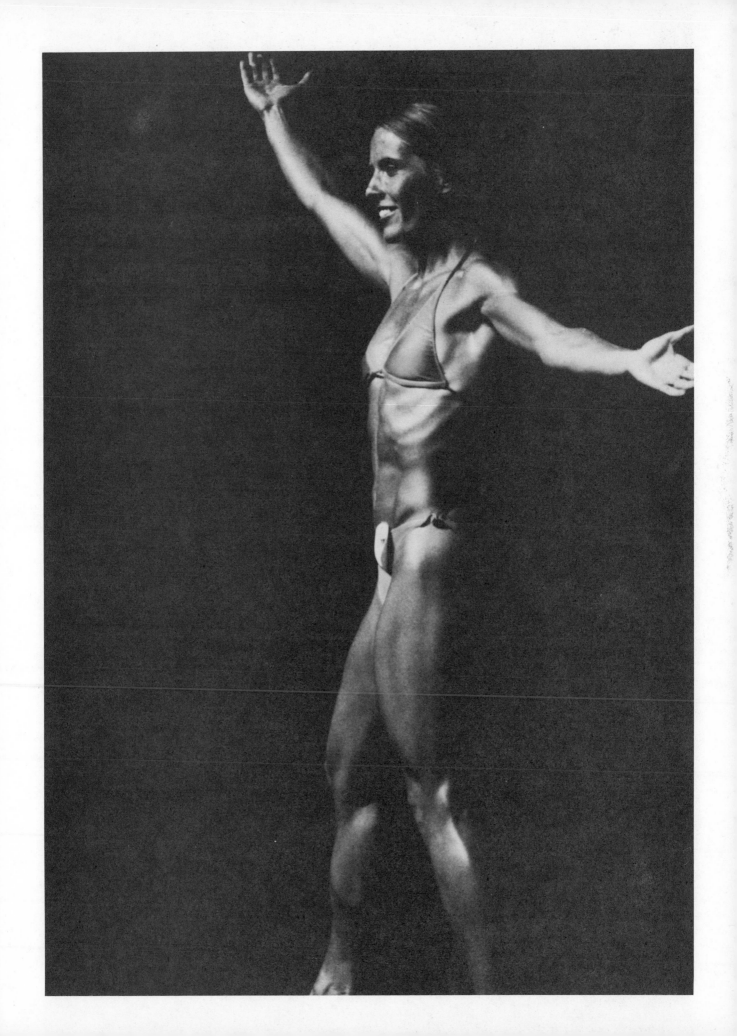

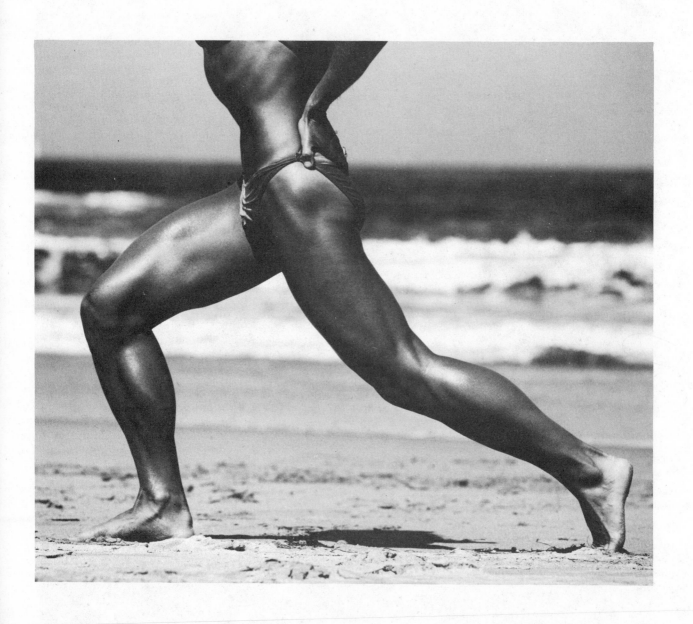

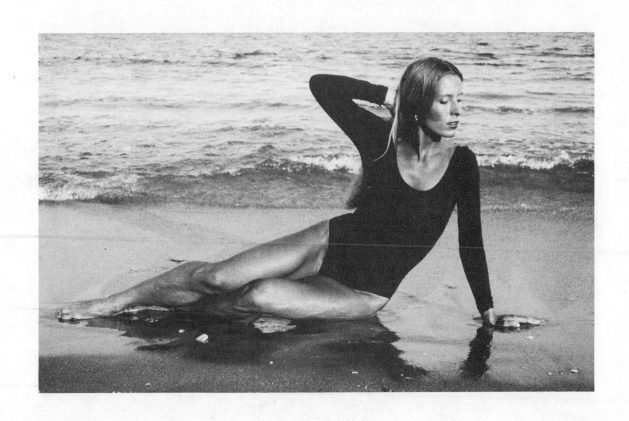

57

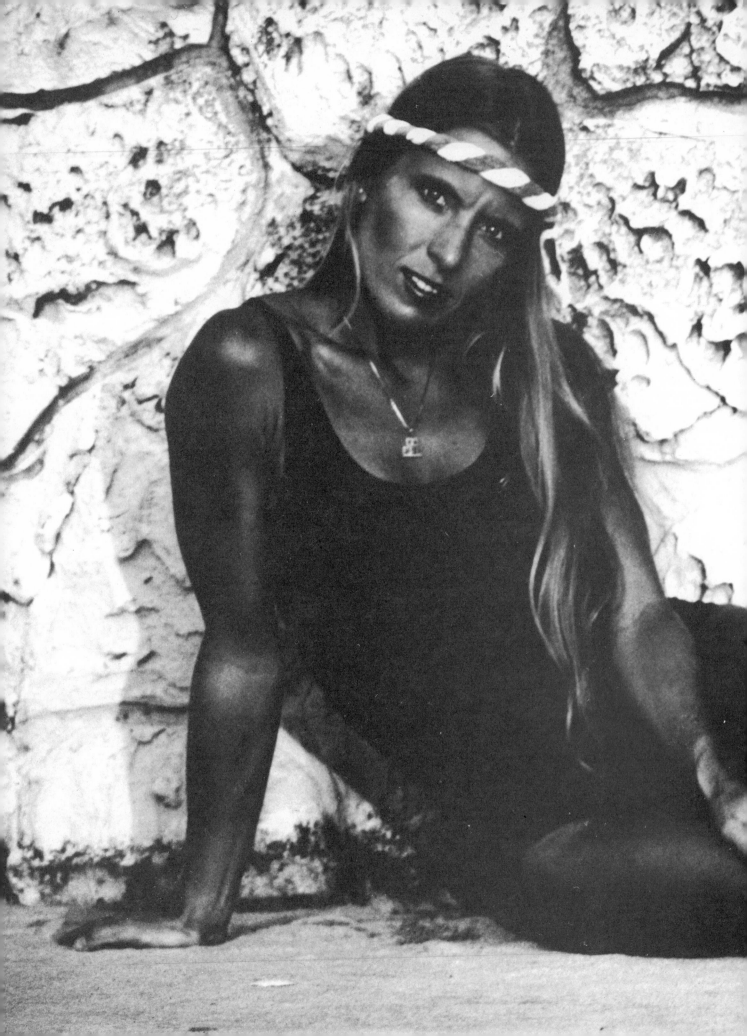

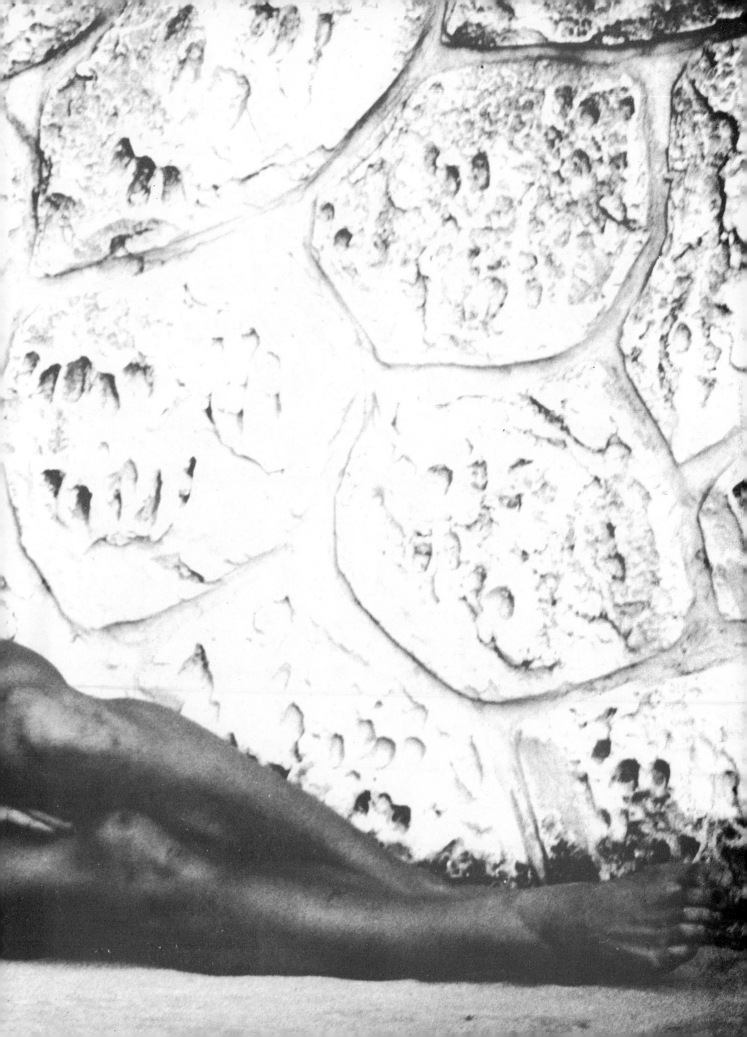

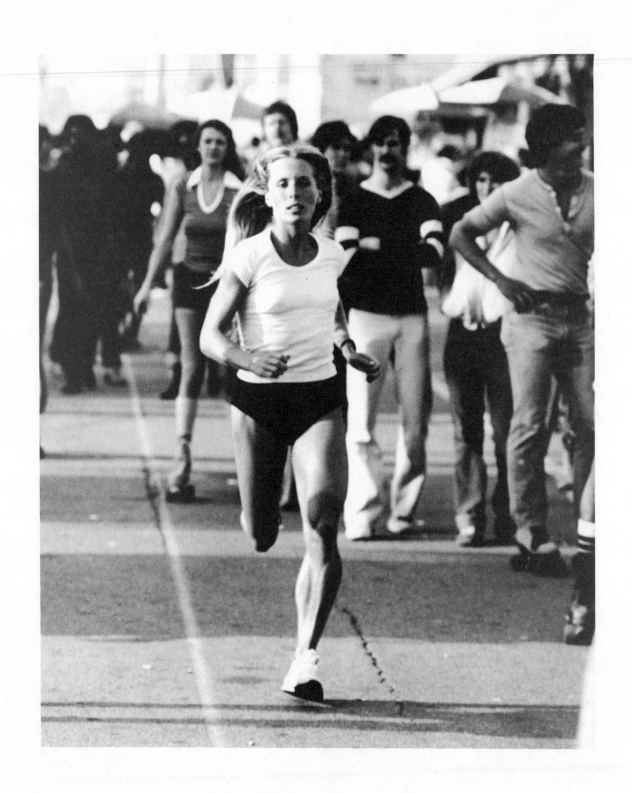

Extracise®

Whether you're training for the Olympic games, or training to fit into your designer jeans, one thing is for sure: that extra effort makes the difference.

That's why I call the type of training program here my special Extracise® plan.

Successive exercises in the plan impose different demands on the body. The training effects upon the heart, lungs, and circulatory system are accumulative, yet flexibility and specific muscular work require you to put forth the extra effort that makes the difference.

And the difference is something you can measure. Keep a chart of your progress with Extracise®. Once you have fully mastered the techniques here and find yourself looking for more of a challenge, do the system using ankle and wrist weights.

What to Expect Now That You're Getting Into Shape

Wouldn't you love to just throw the bathroom scale right out the window? I mean how many times a week can you say "It's not me—the scale must be broken?"

You've always wanted to get into shape, and now that you're doing it, getting rid of the scale is actually not such a bad idea. Because what matters is really how many of your pounds are fat pounds—or, what percentage of your total body weight is fat.

And appearances can be very deceptive. Most people would think of a marathon runner as having less fat than a muscular professional football player because he/she looks thinner. Yet the football player could outweigh the marathon runner by as much as fifty pounds and still have the same percentage of body fat.

It is actually even possible to stay at the same weight while losing fat through exercising. This is because a pound of muscle takes up less room than a pound of fat, so you'll look thinner and lose inches without necessarily losing weight. Just beware, because it does take a long time to gain muscle pounds. Be honest with yourself.

The key to it all is how you feel. You don't need to go to a spa or a sports-medicine institute to have your fat measured with fancy skinfold calipers. You don't really even need your bathroom scale. Because being in shape means that your body and mind are coordinated. Being in shape shows that you have self-respect as well as the right number of inches in the right places. Do you really need to weigh yourself every day now? Aren't there other signs that are just as telling for you—like when you start having trouble doing up the waistband on your designer jeans? Like when you realize that you're still eating and you're no longer hungry? This is proof enough of whether or not your habits need to be changed for the better. You are naturally a person who will make the better choices for yourself.

But before you DO make a frisbee out of your bathroom scale—keep this in mind. You yourself know when you have gained some fat pounds. What to do? Very simple. Begin to eat less. To do this, cut 200 to 300 calories a day from your food intake. If you exercise as well, this could mean a loss of one fat pound or more every week. And this is the way to make sure it stays off.

Remember, fad diets last only as long as the fad. So DO stick with it. The compliments from your friends and neighbors will be nice, but more importantly, you will feel great about yourself—you'll be happy inside your own skin.

And because you've put forth the extra effort, it'll make all the difference.

Okay, now you can get rid of the scale—or at least relegate it to the hall closet. Listen now to what your body is telling you. It's not always saying "FEED ME, FEED ME." Listen for the part where it says, "Hey—what a great team we are."

And that's one of the most memorable aspects of getting into shape.

How Much Is Too Much

Experts agree that the upper limit of body fat for men should not exceed 15 percent. For women, 22 percent is considered to be the upper level. Male athletes in excellent condition should not have more than 7 percent body fat, female athletes not more than 15 percent. The body fat of world-class marathon runners and cross country skiers can range from 3 to 6 percent.

Equipment Needed

- a jump rope.
- a chinning bar—a kid's playground can provide this for you. Portable bars that can fit in any doorway are inexpensive and available at sporting goods stores.
- a strong solid box, bench, or even a cement wall 18–24 inches high.

How Much

The Extracise® plan should take approximately twenty minutes. At first you may only be able to do one minute of certain activities—like jumping rope, for instance. That's okay. Listen to your body. Give enough energy to raise the activities above a mediocre level of output, but be realistic.

How Often

Naturally, how often depends upon the intensity. The general rule is that four workouts per week are better than three, and that five are better than four. If you can only exercise three times a week, increase the length of each session by ten minutes or more, and do the workouts on alternate days.

The absolute minimum is ten minutes of aerobic activity per day. Twenty minutes five times a week of **honest** aerobic activity is considered to be good. Of course, this will not get you into the world championships, but it will maintain your shape. Spend a few minutes before your workout by doing some easy activity as a warm-up, and a few minutes at the conclusion of the workout as a cool-down.

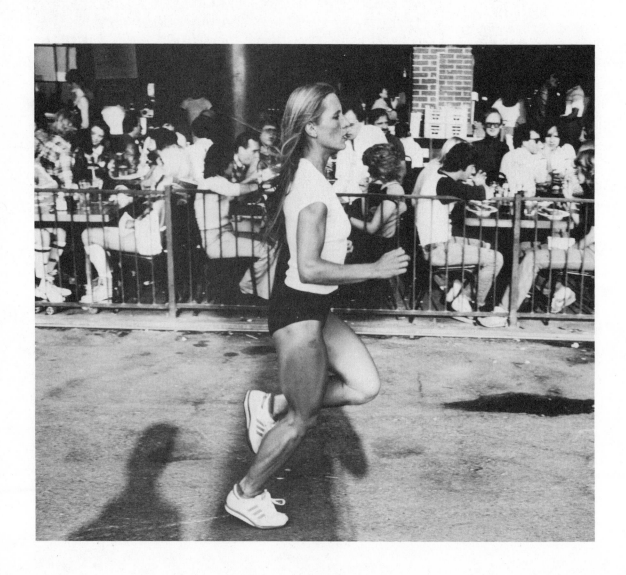

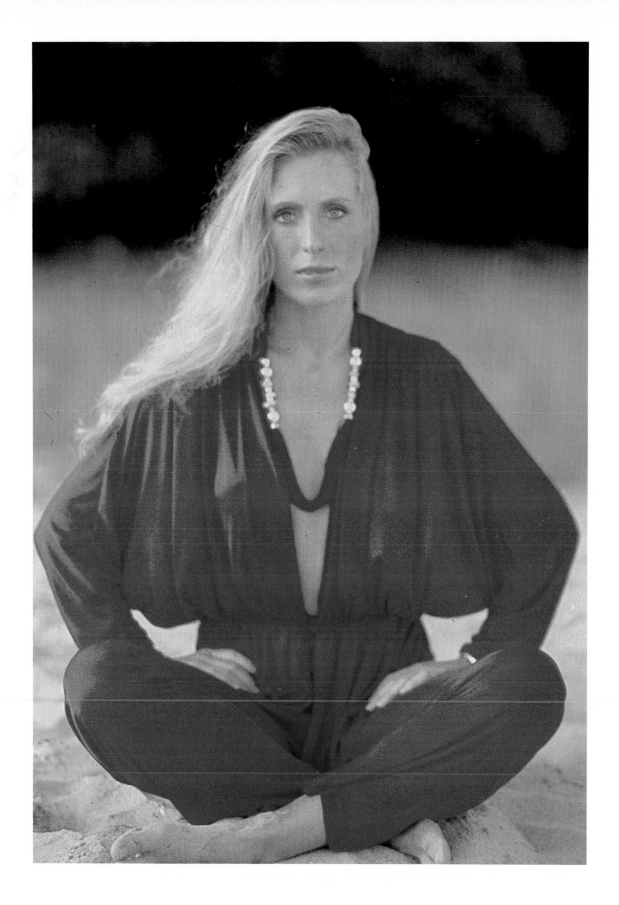

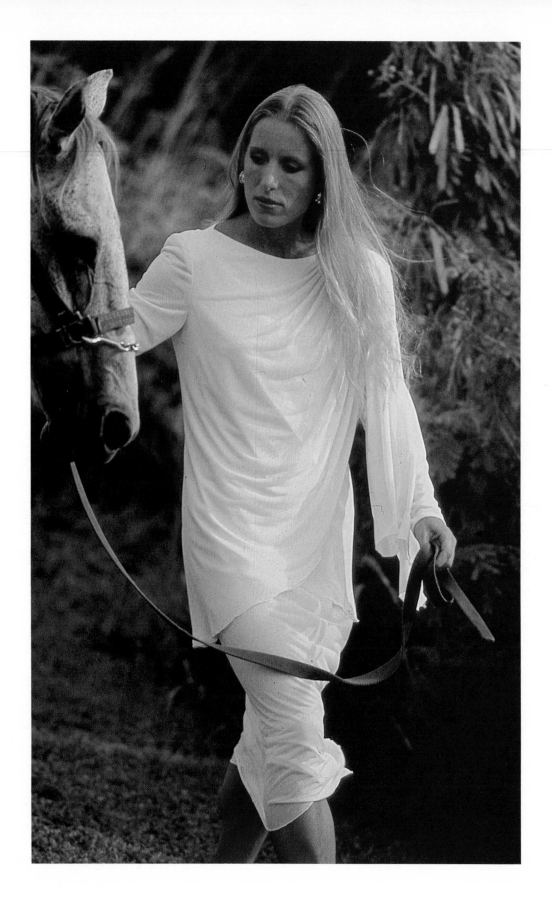

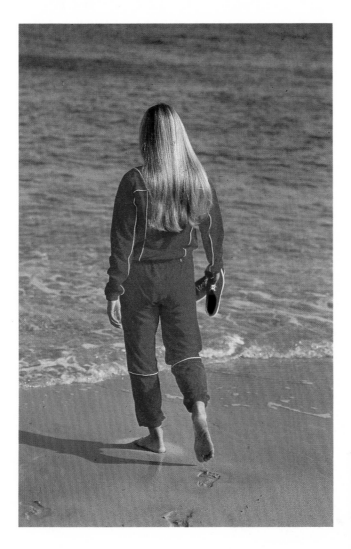
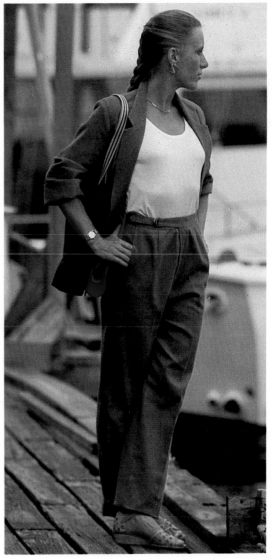

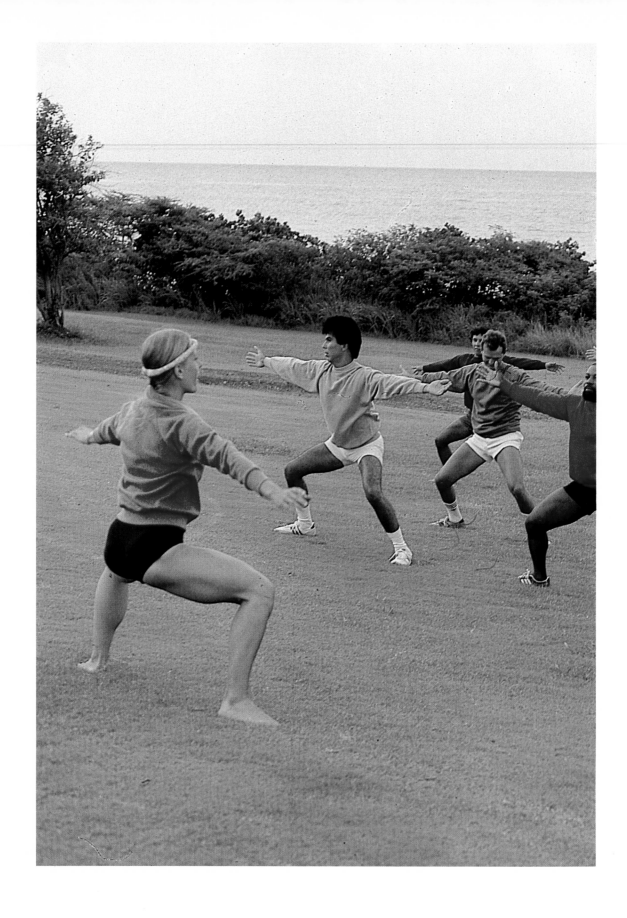

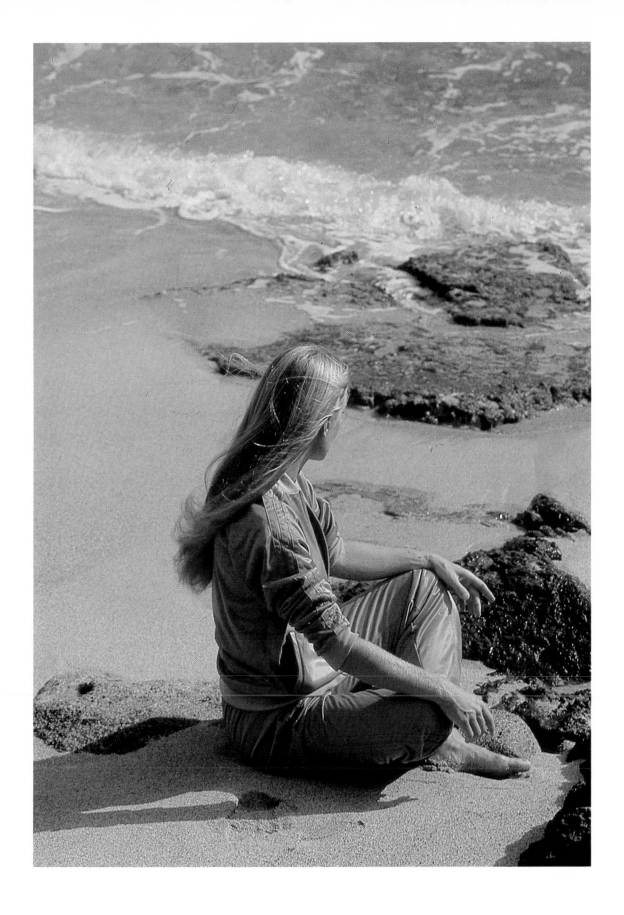

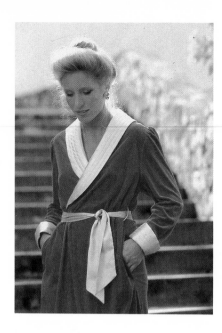

The creatures on our planet—the birds, the animals, the fish, the insects—they do not worry about the purpose of life. For them, the purpose of life is life itself.

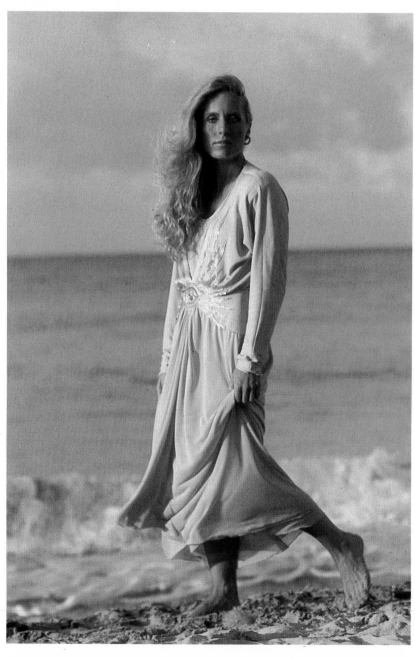

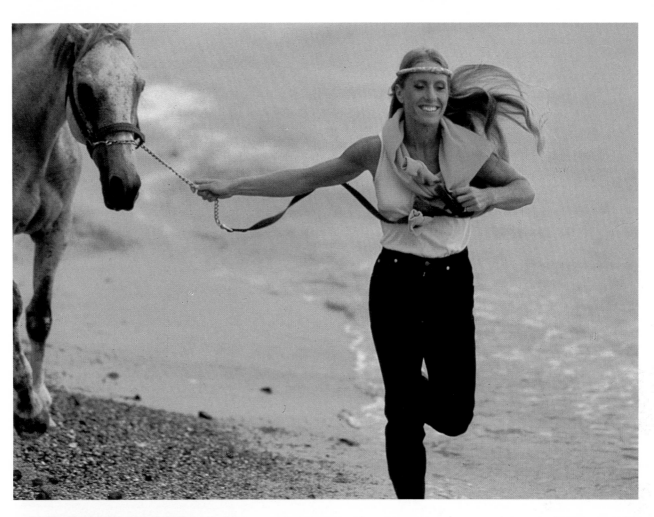

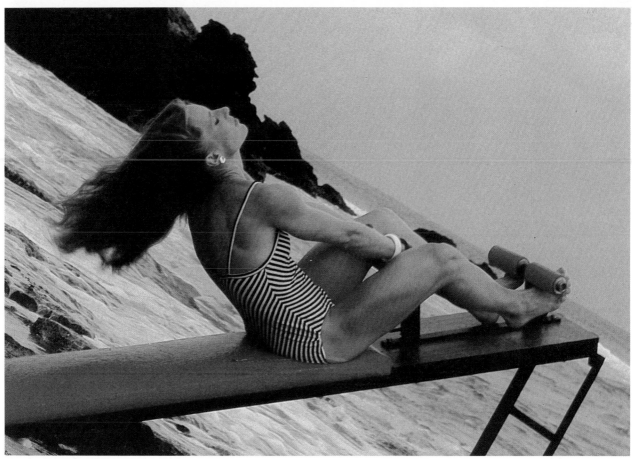

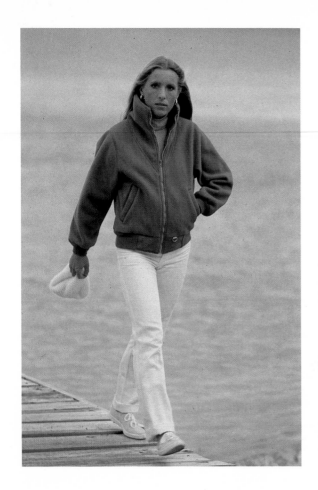
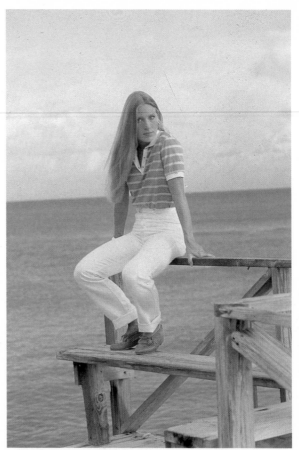
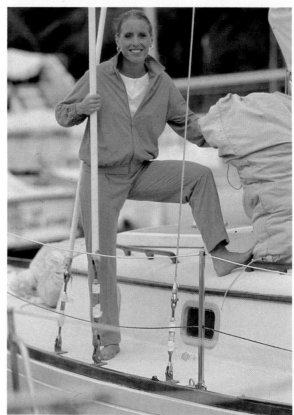

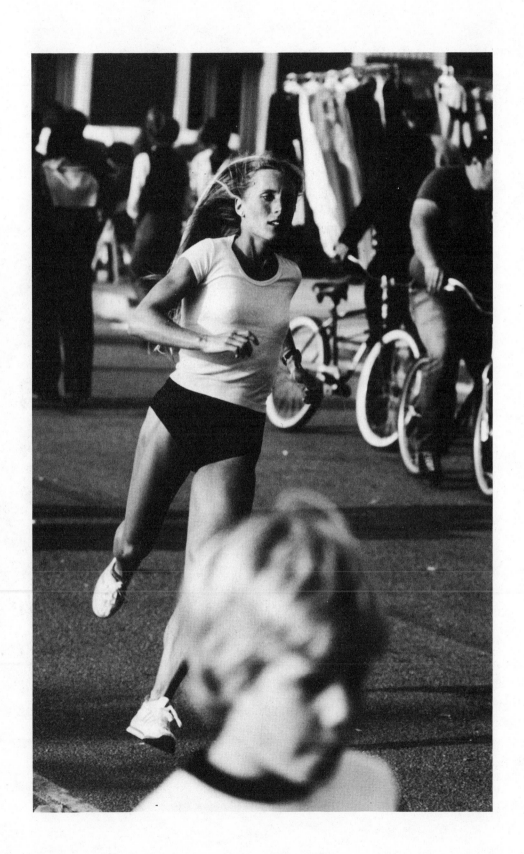

Making Time

1. Set a regular time for your exercise and let nothing keep you from this appointment.
2. Find a workout partner if possible. It is more fun, and it's harder to cancel when someone else is depending on you.
3. Use good equipment. A beautiful leotard and super-comfortable shoes also make you feel good.

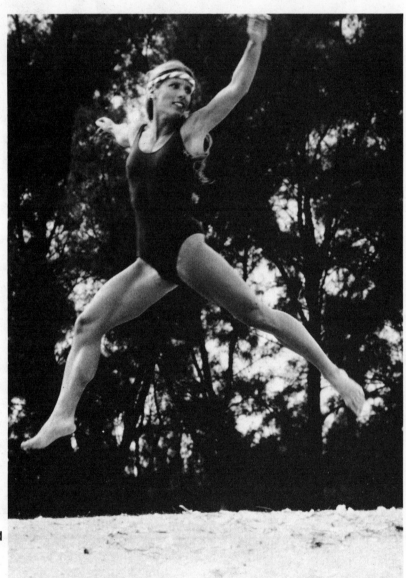

Dreams of freedom that never end —and the place to dream them— the luxury of tropical sun, in an endless blue sky

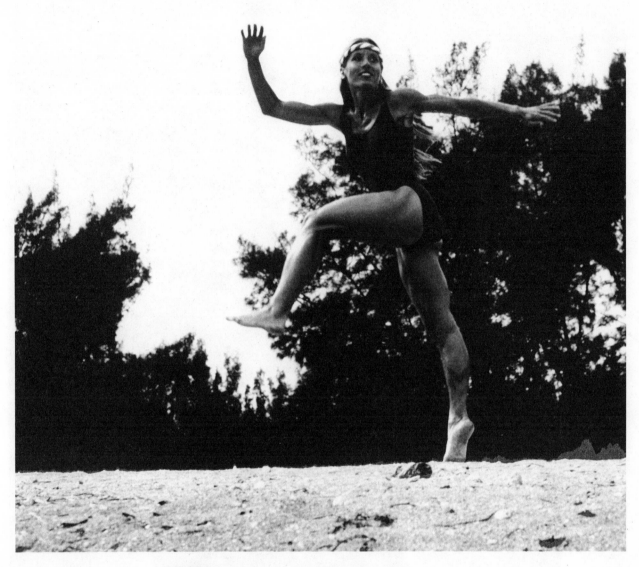

Notes

- Try hard and keep good form.

- Don't rest in between repetitions—return to the starting position and keep the momentum by repeating the movement.

- Move right into the next exercise within ten seconds. Don't waste time on the floor thinking about it.

- Each day, try to do more, even if it's only one rep more.

- Never exercise in sharp pain. This is a test of athletics, not heroics. Of course, your muscles may be "workout-sore"—this is a good hurt. Sharp pain should never be ignored.

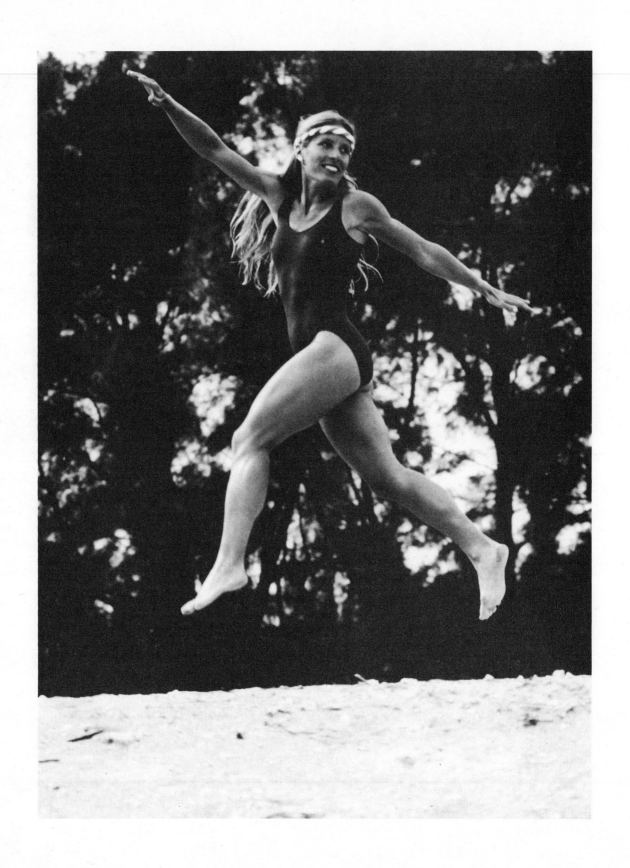

Extracise® Program

1. **Shoulder Shrugs and Circles** _____

   Purpose—Relieves tension in the neck. Uses trapezius muscles.

   Movement—Rotate both shoulders forward, back, and up in a circular motion. Repeat in other direction.

   Goal—Ten in each direction.

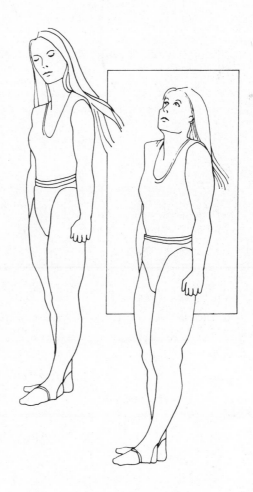

2. Arm Circles

Purpose—Relieves tension in neck and shoulders, and uses the deltoid muscles.

Movement—Make full arm circles in each direction.

Goal—Ten in each direction.

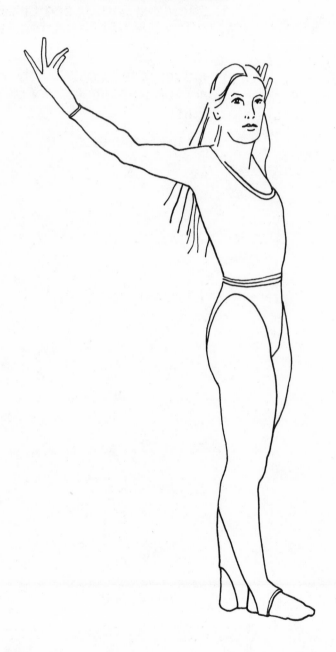

3. Knee to Chest

Purpose—Strengthens the abdominals.

Starting Position—Hang from bar, palms facing away.

Movement—Legs together, bring your knees up toward your chest. Lower and repeat.

Goal—Beginners, five.
Advanced, fifteen.

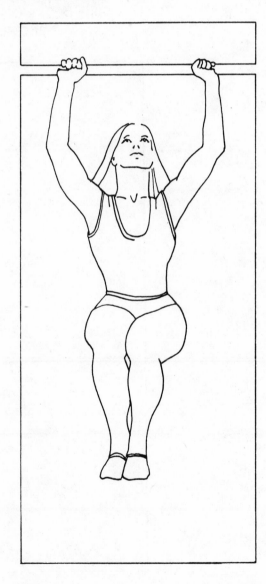

4. Jumping Jacks

Purpose—Primarily aerobic. Uses the legs, arms, and strengthens general coordination.

Starting Position—Hands at side, feet together.

Movement—Jump up, spreading legs and opening arms at the same time, so that your hands touch over your head, arms extended. Then jump, bringing body back to starting position.

Goal—Beginners, one minute.
Advanced, three minutes.

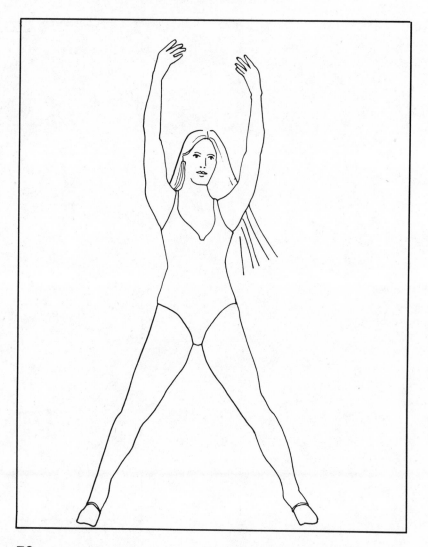

5. Hamstring Stretch with Stool

Purpose—To stretch the back of the leg.

Movement—As shown. Press the leg down. Then relax and bend forward for the stretch. Repeat with other leg.

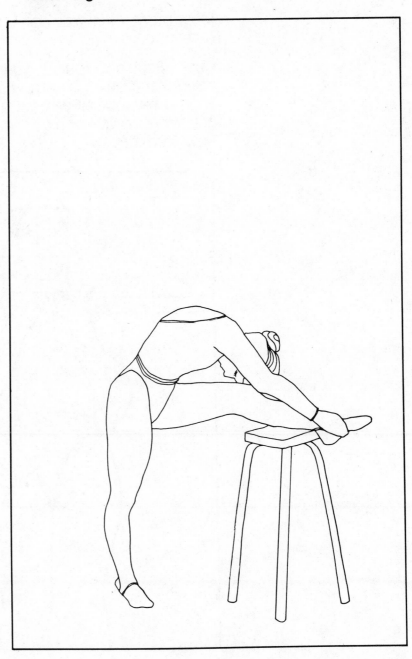

6. Chin-Ups

Purpose—Uses inner chest, biceps.

Starting Position—Close grip, palms facing in for inner chest. Palms facing in, wide grip for outer chest.

Movement—Pull your chin up to the bar. Lower and repeat.

Goal—Beginner, four. If you can't do one, use a chair. Stand on chair with your chin up to the bar. Then lower yourself without using the chair. As you get stronger, you won't need the chair.
Advanced, ten.

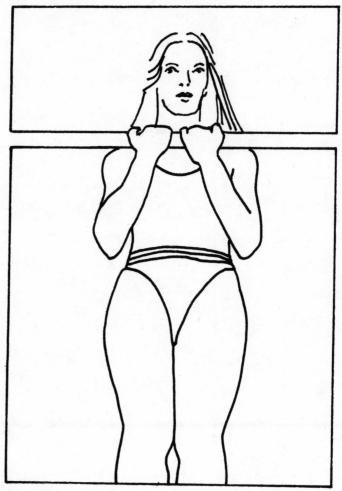

7. Jump Rope _____

Purpose—Primarily aerobic. Uses your legs, arms, and shoulders. Develops coordination.

Goal—Beginners, one minute at a good pace. Advanced, five minutes (120 skips/minute).

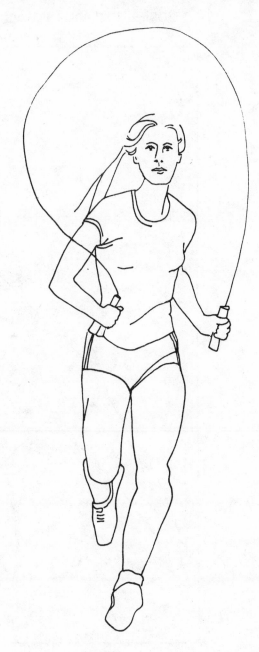

8. Wall Push

Purpose—Stretches the calf muscles.

Movement—With the back leg straight, put heel to the floor. Then, keeping heel on the floor, bend the knee of your front leg.

Goal—Hold for a slow count of fifteen for each leg.

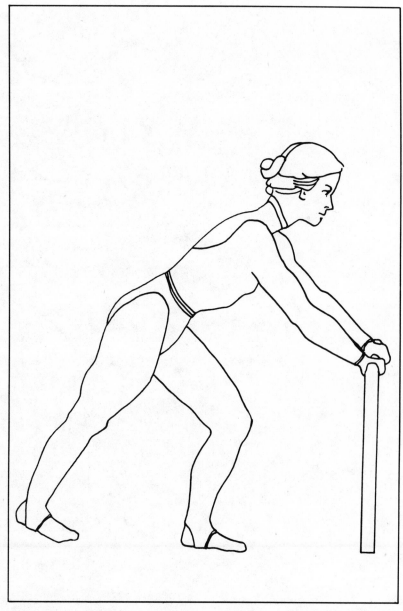

9. Tricep Dips

Purpose—Uses triceps and shoulders.

Starting Position—Feet on floor, resting on heels. Hands on bench or chair as shown.

Movement—Extend arms, but do not lock elbows at the top position. Lower yourself and repeat.

Goal—Beginners, ten.
　　　　Advanced, thirty.

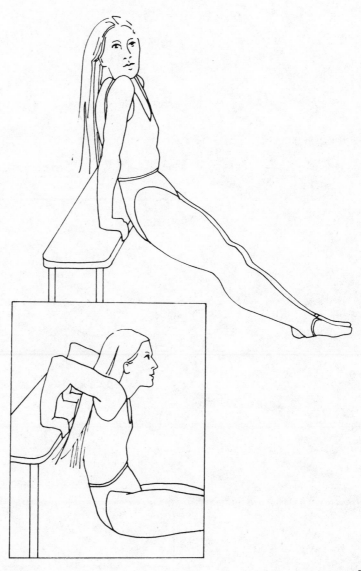

10. **Side Karate Stretch** _____

Purpose—Develops balance and stretches the groin and ankle areas.

Starting Position—Keep the heels of both feet on the floor. As you become more flexible, move your feet wider apart. Repeat for other leg.

Goal—Hold for a slow fifteen count.

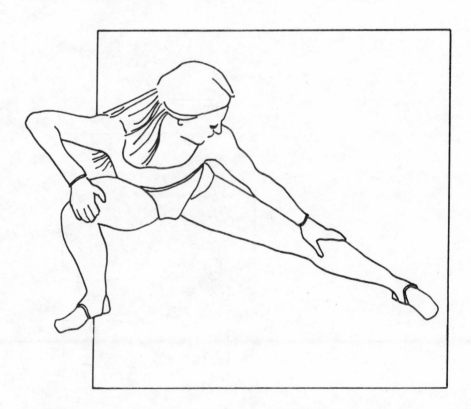

11. Step-Ups

Purpose—Primarily aerobic. Also has a great strengthening potential for the thighs, hamstring, and derriere.

Starting Position—Stand in front of a wall or box 18–24 inches in height, feet together.

Movement—Put one foot on top of box, then step up with other foot. Step down with first foot. Repeat. Then alternate what is the first foot.

Goal—Beginners, ten times each foot.
Advanced, twenty times each foot.

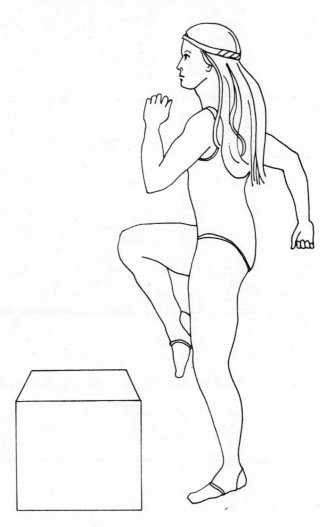

12. Push-Ups

Purpose—Uses the chest and triceps.

Starting Position—Lie facedown on the floor, with your weight supported by the hands and toes.

Hands 6 inches apart—works inner chest and triceps.
Hands 24 inches apart—works midchest and shoulders.
Hands 36 inches apart—outer chest, shoulders, and latissimus dorsi (back).

Movement—Push the arms straight while keeping the body rigid. Lower slowly and repeat.

Goal—Beginners, ten. Start with whatever you can do, keeping good form. One perfect push-up is good.
Advanced, thirty.

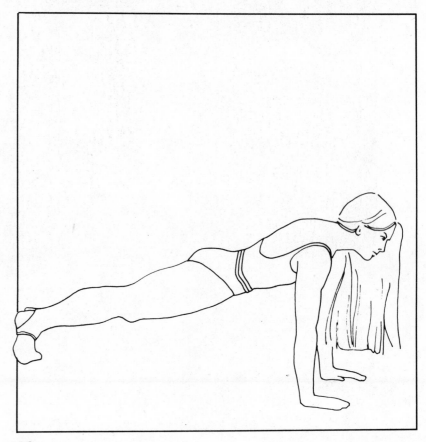

13. Bent-Over Leg Raise

Purpose—Strengthens derriere (gluteus maximus) and back of thighs (hamstrings).

Starting Position—Bend at the waist from a standing position, resting hands on the floor and keeping both legs straight.

Movement—Keeping leg straight, lift one leg straight back and up high, flexing foot. Keep knee pointed at floor, head lowered. Don't arch back. Only your leg should move up and back. Hips, head, back stay level. Repeat with other leg.

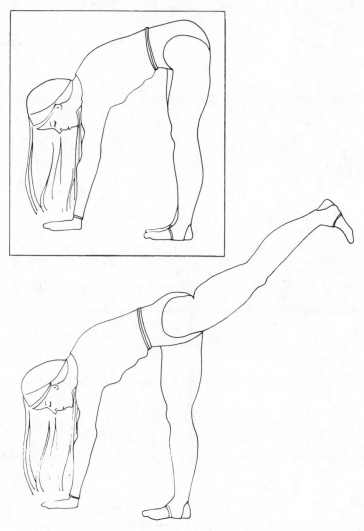

14. The Horse

Purpose—Uses the thighs and your willpower.

Starting Position—Feet apart slightly wider than shoulder width. Back straight. Knees bent as shown.

Movement—None. Just stay there as long as you can. Time the effort, trying to increase time with each session.

Goal—Beginners, one minute.
　　　　Advanced, five minutes.

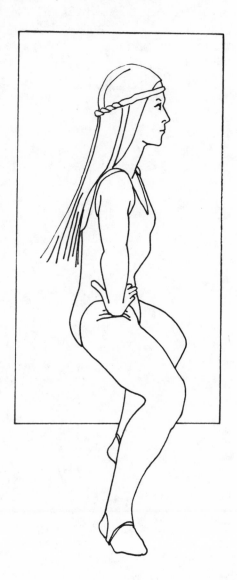

15. Running Kickbacks

Purpose—Aerobic. Also works the back of the thigh (hamstrings).

Movement—Your heels will actually be lightly kicking your derriere as you perform the exercise. Think of keeping your thighs in a straight line—not allowing the knee to pass the imaginary vertical line from your nose to your toes. Proceed forward in this stylized running form. Count one step each time your starting foot touches the ground (e.g., your right foot).

Goal—Beginners, fifty steps.
       Advanced, one hundred steps.

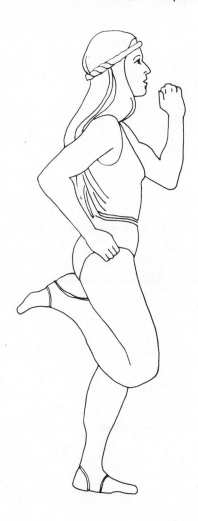

16. Arm Circles _____
See exercise 2.

17. Hamstring Stretch _____
See exercise 5.

18. Salute to Sun _____
Purpose—Stretches legs, arms, chest, and abdomen.

Starting Position—As shown. Hold for a slow fifteen count. Switch legs and repeat.

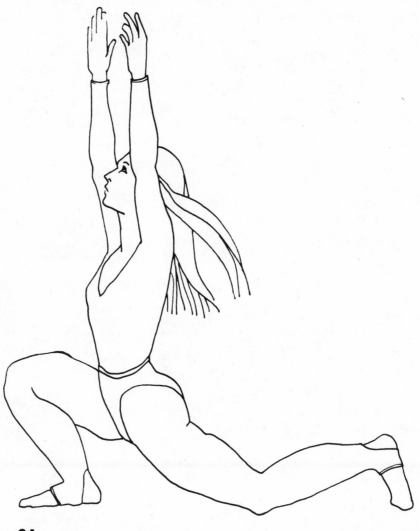

19. Frog Sit

Purpose—To stretch inner thighs, feet, and ankles.

Starting Position—Foot soles together. The object is to bring the heels close to the body while keeping the knees close to the floor. Keep your back straight and inhale deeply. Exhale fully and repeat five to ten times.

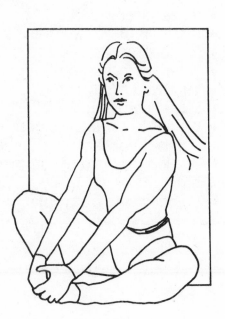

The New You

- A better shape—a sleeker body
- No inhibitions about your body
- Better posture
- Everyday problems will not be as much of a hassle
- More vitality
- Self-respect
- Better sleep
- Better immunity to disease
- A coordinated mind and body
- The right inches in the right places
- Improved circulation
- More energy for work
- Weight loss if overweight
- You look forward to each new day
- You look forward to summer, and wearing your teenie bikini
- Compliments from your friends

Questions and Answers

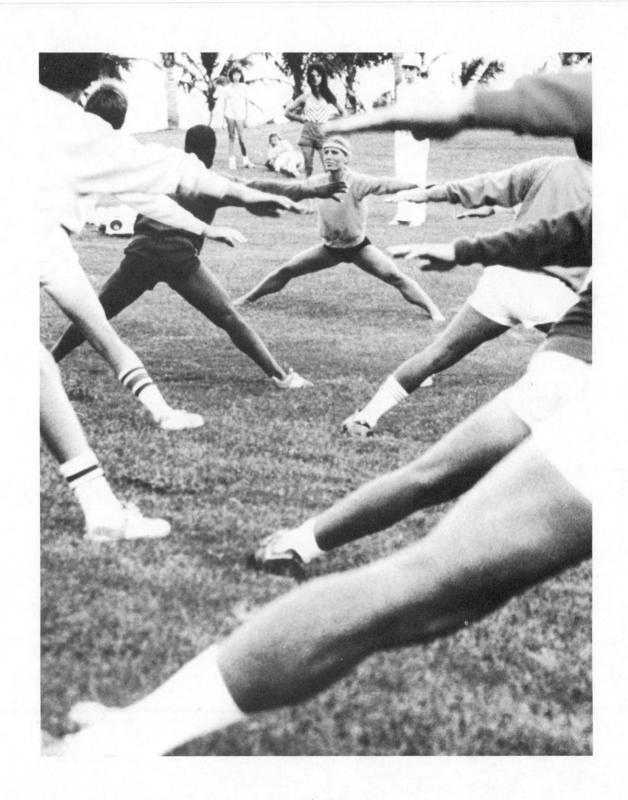

Questions and Answers

Q. What is the best exercise for losing weight?

A. The best exercise of all is very simple. It's called "Pushing Yourself Away from the Table."

Q. All my life I've been the quintessential klutz. I seem to have been born pudgy, and stayed that way. I've tried to diet a million times, but before long I end up bingeing on a fudge ripple or whatever else is handy. In high school I was dumpy, and ten years later I'm still dumpy. Any suggestions?

A. Let go of the picture of yourself you had as an adolescent. Perhaps there was a time when you convinced yourself that comfort was to be found in those quarts of fudge ripple. Why turn your shape or size, or whatever makes you feel less than perfect, into a way of life?

Regardless of your childhood circumstances, environment, or anything else that we blame things on, keep in mind just one thing: You have free will. So instead of sitting around waiting for real and imagined disasters to strike, use your free will to make some right choices for yourself—today.

Are you letting little voices from the past get air time in your present? Whenever we hear one of those voices telling us how unattractive or stupid we are, we must stop it immediately and divert our attention. Get up and do some push-ups at two o'clock in the morning, if that's what it takes.

Finally, ask yourself, "What am I getting out of reliving past scenarios that should be forgotten?" Are you still trying to "pay" for the mistake with the resultant guilt you feel every time the old scenes are played back in your mind? Are you still thinking of the perfect

89

stinging invectives you wish you had said? Are you still trying to even the score?

Live freely in the present. Do that by dismissing the past, not merely by saying "I must forget; I must forget." That will only make you even more conscious of remembering. Dismiss the past by diverting yourself from it, by focusing your life energy on improving yourself from this moment on.

You are naturally a person who knows how to make good choices. We all have that innate ability, but simply don't use it at times.

Be here, right now. Wake up in the morning and take a deep, deep breath, and feel fresh and clean and ready to use that free will of yours to do your best, right now.

Q. **Is there anything you can do when traveling to prevent the kind of body stiffness you feel at the end of a long flight? Come to think of it, I commute forty-five minutes every day just to get to work. By the time I get there at 9:00 A.M., my body already feels steamrollered. Help!**

A. Relaxed, comfortable travel really is possible. I'm almost constantly on the road, so over the years I've developed some exercises that can be done even with the seat belt fastened. And no one ever realizes that I'm actually exercising on board. Here are a few of my favorites:

1. Push down hard on the armrests with your elbows. Make your shoulders push down as hard as you can. Hold for a slow count of ten while breathing deeply.

2. Squeeze your buttocks together as hard as you can. Also tense each and every muscle in your legs. Hold for a slow ten count while breathing deeply.

3. Hug yourself. Let your head drop forward and pull slowly but firmly on your shoulders. This really stretches the muscles between your shoulder blades.

4. Pretend to adjust the light or air vent while remain-

90

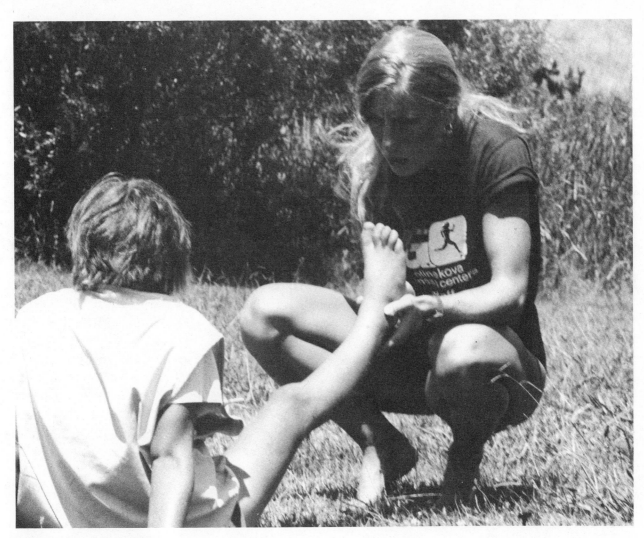

Helping a young athlete with an old cure—mud on a beesting

ing seated. Alternate arms and inhale as you lift each arm up.

5. Slip your shoes off. Curl up your toes, and then stretch them out as far as possible. Repeat fifty times. Try to extend your legs from the knees if at all possible.

6. Above all, remember to relax and keep a positive attitude. Flying past those cloud cities in the sky is a good time to count your blessings—even to create some happy fantasies.

Remain calm when driving to work, even if you get stuck in a traffic jam. It's a good time to be glad thay you have a job to drive to. That kind of happy thinking can lead to all kinds of imaginings. The sky's the limit—and you'll arrive intact, and smiling.

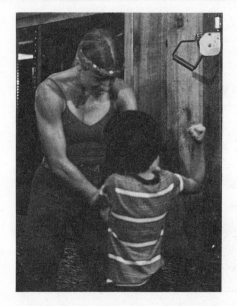

Q. What can you do about job stress? I just feel burnt-out from my job, which is high intensity beyond belief right now.

A. Physical activity has the power to defuse us—to transform stress; it is the intrinsic factor in sparing ourselves "burnout."

Vigorous activity—the stuff that makes your heart go pit-a-pat—allows you to let go of all the insignificant and even irritating events of the day, and thereby find calmness. Our minds require the activity from our bodies in order to release energy and feel inner peacefulness.

We can also use fitness to change old ways of thinking about ourselves and others. Through exercise we can learn to accept ourselves. The daily reality of charging down the home stretch at your own best pace can transfer its meaning and satisfaction to other areas in your life.

And my success in business has proven definitively to me that tenacity learned through extending your limits athletically is thoroughly transferable to the boardroom.

When you feel good about yourself, it shows in direct proportion to your productivity. By definition, without any stress at all we'd technically be dead. The trick is to learn how to defuse the negative stress and create the by-products of strength and endurance . . . and thus more energy. The body and mind are meant to function as a unit, and exercise is the unifying force.

Q. What makes muscles grow?

A. There must be stimulation inside the body itself. This means exercise. Then there must be nutrients available for the stimulated muscle cells to grow.

Technically, the chemical reactions at the cellular level of the body are quite complex. It works like this: The intense contracting of the muscle causes production of **creatin** in the muscle fiber, which in turn causes an increase of a substance **myosin**, which

92

in turn enables the fiber to produce stronger contractions.

Then the whole cycle repeats. More intense contractions by exercise create more creatin and the muscle produces more myosin, and then it's back to the beginning of the cycle again. But growth is stimulated through exercise (intense contracting of the muscles) and the rest follows.

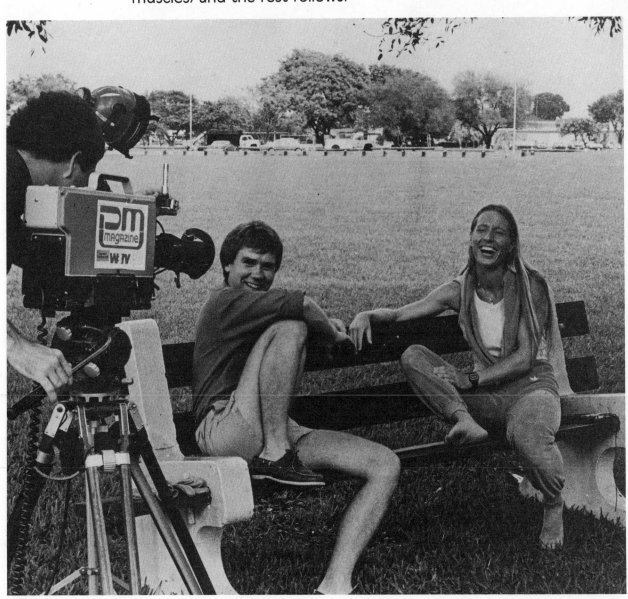

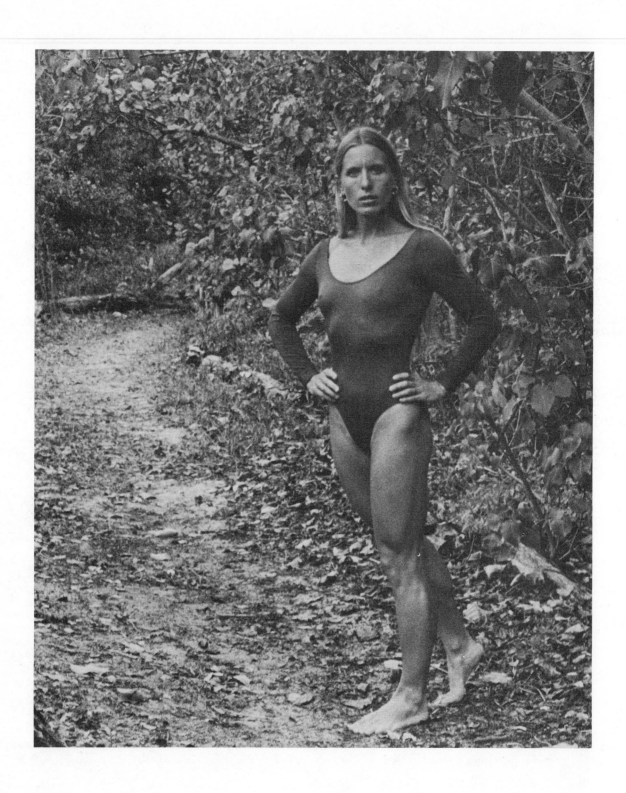

Q. Is aging the ultimate fear for an athlete?

A. I come from a hearty family where you don't receive any deference because of age, or any seniority points until you reach your early nineties.

I know a person can remain strong and vital all of his/her life. The time you spend on fitness in your twenties, thirties, and forties is like an investment in the bank that you can draw on in your seventies, eighties, and nineties.

I have done physical work since I was a child—carrying a stack of newspapers on my shoulders and trudging through the snow to deliver them, for example.

As a teenager, I was a member of many national teams as a sprinter. The only difference between the workouts I did then, and what I do now as a marathoner, is that now I do five times as much.

Personally, I welcome the years. Living a healthy, natural life without drugs, and obeying nature's laws, has allowed me over fifteen years of competition on the international level, and I know that I have yet to peak.

It's been said before, but in athletics I can vouch for the statement: "You're not getting older, you're getting better."

I intend to be the fittest ninety-five-year-old on my block!

Q. Please give me some advice. I've always been what is tactfully called "a full-figured woman." I recently decided to drop a few pounds (like about twenty pounds), but my boyfriend seems pretty resistant to the idea. He says, "I like my woman to be soft and fleshy."

A. I would have to answer your question by asking another question.

How could any man, in the name of love, want

his woman to be something we know to be unhealthy? For his pleasure?

Women are finding out that strength is beauty. That the addition of sleek muscle and sinew to the body adds to her naturally feminine physique. Firm muscle tone can only accentuate your already existing curves.

Think of a ballerina—sweeping her foot off the ground and over her head in one movement. One of the most graceful in dance, that move takes sheer power to achieve. Just try it.

In the meantime, my advice is to get in shape. If your boyfriend truly loves you, he will be happy for your achievements as you improve yourself.

However, if someone that close to you could be so threatened by your wanting to be healthy, sleek, and strong, perhaps it's time to reevaluate your relationship.

Q. Do you have to have big muscles to be strong?

A. No. I've often seen relatively small athletes outlift and outrun their big brawny teammates.

Leverage, angles of the body, skill, and training are only a few of the many factors involved. And let's not forget motivation. There are remarkable feats of strength documented—such as the one-hundred-three-pound housewife who lifted up the front end of the family station wagon in order to free her baby.

Q. What is a typical daily Olinekova workout schedule?

A. Interviewers often ask me for a typical daily workout, but this is just impossible. Some days I do three or four workouts. Some days I don't run at all, but may walk for a few hours. Other days I'll get up, fling myself out the door and run as far as I can, as fast as I can. The workouts are rarely duplicated, and there are no "typical" weeks. This is because after more than fifteen years as a competitive athlete, I have learned how to

96

listen to my body and train instinctively. I've learned to take days off after extraordinary efforts, and also use rope jumping, dancing, cycling, and other activities to work my heart.

Running is the least difficult part of my workouts these days, yet I'm running faster and recovering more quickly than I did as a teenager. My twenty-mile runs are now the easiest of my exercises.

Perhaps my mind is becoming better trained. I'd been holding back given my potential, it seems, according to scientific findings in the laboratory. Now I just let my body do what it feels—no strings, no restraints. Just the letting go, that exquisite feeling in its power—a low burning explosion of breathless abandonment.

Q. But what about discipline and determination?

A. Reporters also often try to peg me with the words "discipline" and "determination." But for me, these words don't even come into it. Activity is my passion. Most of all, I think I'm driven simply by a heart that yearns for the immense and nourishing idea of personal freedom, which for me comes from running up the side of a mountain, breaking a finish tape, lifting weights, dancing, or any one of a hundred things that allow me to go beyond the peripheries.

Discipline? More like addiction, I think.

Q. Do you have a personal stress-relieving formula?

A. Living on an island has many pleasures for me, but one of them is to be constantly surrounded by and aware of the power of the ocean. Many times after a hard workout I've stood on a "thinking rock" in order to resolve a problem, only to realize, after a very short time of watching the turquoise water, that my problem is really no more than a single ripple on the surface of the ocean.

The mundane things seem like such trifles then.

97

In scuba diving, I've learned how calm the lower depths of the ocean can be, even when the surface water is virtually frothing with activity.

I feel that way myself sometimes—the more furious the sprint, the calmer I feel inwardly, the more intact, because my body is meeting with its own reality and allowing my mind to fuel this strength of action with inner calm.

So when the endless phone calls, the tough negotiations, and the constant business of doing business begins to pile up, I literally run out of the office and stage a furious workout. It works every time.

Q. Is it possible to ''spot reduce''?

A. No. While controlling food intake, fat is metabolized out of fat cells all over the body. This process is indiscriminate.

Exercise focusing on specific areas of the body can improve the **tone** of the muscle under the fat. In the abdominal area, for instance, loss of inches of the girth may result from an intense abdominal program involving sit-ups and the like.

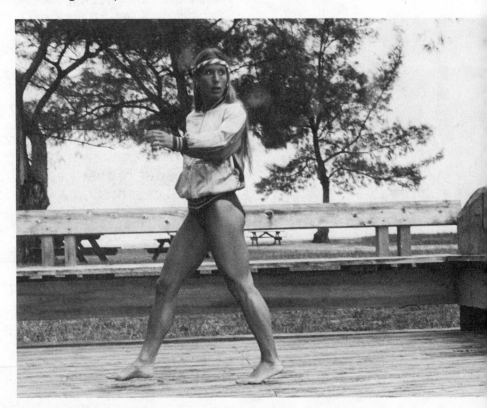

This loss actually occurs, however, because the abdominal muscles are now able to better perform the task of holding your entrails in place. You still have to work the fat off by controlling excess eating and exercising to burn off the stored fat that is already there.

Q. What about vibrating belts? Can you lose weight from them?

A. Mechanical vibrating belts (I call them ''fat jigglers'') can be relaxing, but fat cannot be vibrated off your body.

Q. How about rubber sweat suits?

A. These outfits are supposed to make you sweat off the fat. Wrong. The weight loss is only temporary dehydration, which is replaced as soon as you drink back the fluid. Body fat has only a small percentage of water, anyway, so passive sweating is not going to affect it.

Q. ''No pain, no gain'' is what I've always heard. Does exercise have to be a ''grit your teeth'' experience to do you any good?

A. You should never exercise in pain. However, the ''pain'' or discomfort of being a little out of breath, or the ''pain'' of waiting a few months for your body to improve—that's something quite different.

As far as exercise being a ''grit your teeth'' experience, any dentist will tell you that grinding your molars (bruxism) is never healthy.

Certainly you have to expect to put out some effort—after all, if it were easy to be in shape, **everyone** would look terrific.

But when the obstacles are too heroic for even a good epic movie, it's time to reevaluate your fitness routine. Fitness should be fun. Find something that can give you the pleasure of accomplishment, then stay with it.

99

If you are in a plus or positive frame of mind and someone calls you a damn fool, you'll just shrug it off and think nothing of it. But if your state of mind is negative, how will you react? Negatively. You'll get angry and irritable. More than likely you'll carry a chip on your shoulder all through the day. Think about it.

"He got out of the wrong side of the bed this morning," we say after watching someone slam the screen door, grouch at the dog, and cut someone else off at the intersection.

The point is that if our energy is positive, then the sky is always blue regardless of whether it's raining or gray. "But there is suffering and pain in life," some will cry. How can a sensitive person be blind to it all and still be a decent human being?

There's more to it than that, and there *is* a way to change your perspective. You can go through life unable to see anything but death and destruction all around you. If you have a positive outlook, however, you can see even death differently.

Death is the currency that makes life valuable and abundant. Death makes the reality of our birth and living even more wonderful. If we lived forever, would time be as precious? If there were no destruction, would creation still be a miracle to us? Even on the most mundane level, this holds true.

Food is a blessing to us when we are hungry. But when we eat out of boredom or frustration or anger, then food becomes a curse because it brings a new unhappiness in the form of obesity and ill health.

The states of lacking and wanting can be gifts if we possess positive energy. There have been times in my life when I was struggling and on a skateboard budget, but being in shape and running down the street made me feel that my body handled like a finely tuned Porsche.

If you think this way, you can find happiness even in the face of negative events.

If you're tired and stuck in traffic on your way to work in the morning, take the opportunity to reflect happily on the fact that you have a job to go to at all.

100

If you become ill or injured, take this heaven-sent chance to rest up and strengthen your spirit. After all, if there is nothing at all that you can do to change the situation, then you must change yourself.

Energize for Success

Each of us has a reserve of strength and energy that we never use. Motivation to achieve is the key phrase here. Remarkable feats of strength have been documented—such as the 103-pound housewife who lifted up the front end of the family station wagon in order to free her baby.

This is *not* magic. This is a demonstration of the positive energy and strength that is within all of us—energy and strength that you can use to succeed.

Much has been said about success. And yet most people don't really understand what it is and how to get the "it" once they figure "it" out. Actually, the formula is quite simple and it goes like this.

DESIRE + ACTION = SUCCESS

First there must be the desire. Let's go back to the housewife: Her instinct as a mother is to want to help her baby. But that alone is not enough to save the child's life. She didn't just stand there screaming and crying that her baby must be saved. She *Acted* upon the desire. She ran over to the car and lifted the thing up and saved the child's life. Mission accomplished. SUCCESS.

But you don't have to wait for a life-threatening situation to occur before you plug into this special positive source of energy. It's always there for you to use—all the time.

Start first thing in the morning. Just as each year has only one New Year's Day, so each day has only one first waking moment.

Begin the day in this moment by taking a deep breath, stretching and infusing your body and mind with vibrant, positive thoughts. Then jump out of bed and get on with it. You've started the day with some desire for it. Now apply some action and go for it.

You *deserve* to have a successful day today.

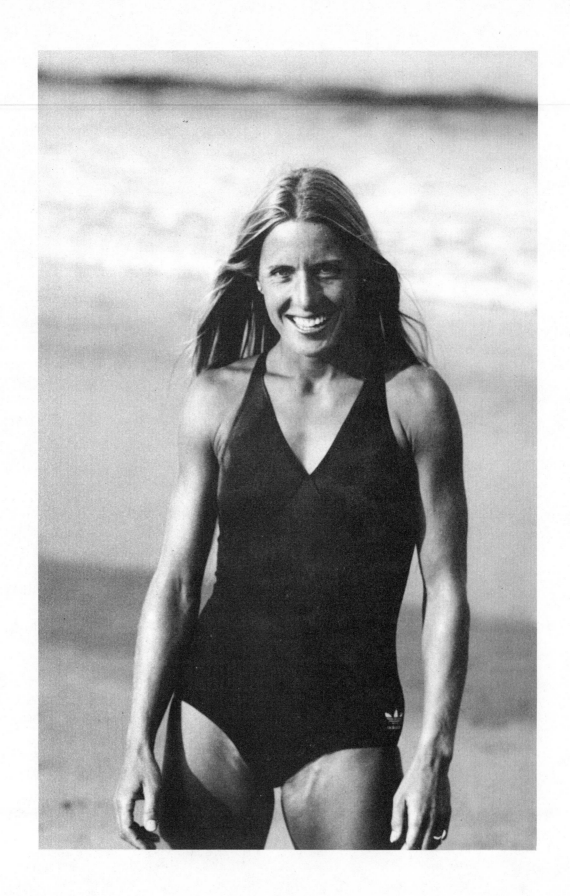

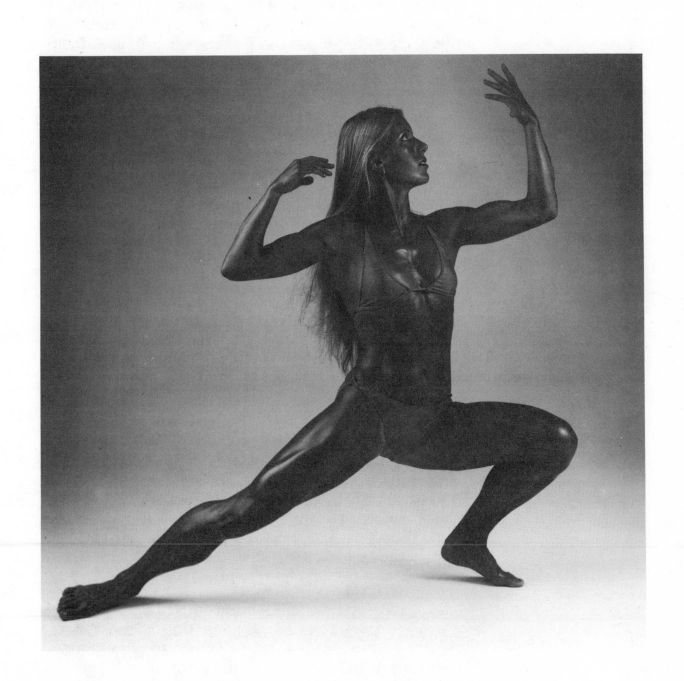

Now apply your energy to make it happen. You can shape your future. You have free will. Use it. Make better choices for yourself. Today monitor your thoughts—throw out the negatives and replace them with positives.

Somebody yells at you. Forget it. "A soft answer turneth away wrath," says the Bible. It's true. If someone is trying to draw you into an argument, they're really trying to vacuum you into negativity. Resist it. Remain calm. Try to see things their way. Leave your emotions out of it and use your logic to solve the problem—your logic, your positive energy. For if you believe there is a solution, you will find it.

"Power Is the Ultimate Aphrodisiac"

This is an oft quoted saying, and it's true in a sense probably never intended. When you have power over your own mind and body, it is very stimulating in every way just to be alive.

You feel happy and secure inside your own skin, and you know why. You have respected yourself enough to become stronger, and it shows. To be vital and alive—that's what sensuality is all about. To be fit is to feel sexy—not necessarily in a Hollywood pin-up sense, but in a lasting way! Sexuality is the creative explorative life force. There is abundant pleasure that you can receive from life as a result of the positive interaction of mind and body. That's undoubtedly the beauty of knowing your own power—the beauty of being able to both give and receive energy in love. If everyone on earth could know the power of this love, then how could war and hate remain for long?

Why shuffle through life too tired to cope when you can stride through life with vitality and strength? Socrates, the famous philosopher of the ancient Greeks, said, "What a disgrace it is for a man to grow without ever seeing the beauty and strength of which his body is capable."

Everyone can get stronger. As the world moves toward harder times, this precious self-mastery takes on increasing significance. In the chaos that we see around

104

us, we need at least to be in complete physical and mental command of ourselves—to have the strength to cope, to remain rational and to retain positive values. This is to have achieved personal freedom.

The positive values derived from fitness are transferable to every other facet of your life. Being fit says a lot about you. It says that you are a person who succeeds today in your fitness program—tomorrow in whatever you aspire to do. You are more aware of the moment, more attuned to the present because you have begun to take care of yourself. You are creating your own future.

That's what positive energy is all about. You have control of your future if you have a strong, positive will. A person who is weak and negative, even if he/she is on the right track, will succeed in nothing and be unable to move forward.

But remember: You cannot expect to achieve a positive will, and to have positive energy without effort—ceaseless effort.

People often complain that the world is a negative, aggressive jungle full of depressing events and people. This is the kind of pessimism that keeps the world from changing. We have to get rid of the idea that any small effort is futile in the face of a vast and unchanging world. Because one light can light a thousand other lights. If nothing else changes in the world other than you—one person—then the world is better by one person. To change the world, you must begin by changing yourself. You have the power to do that and you *can* do it if you kindle the extra effort that makes the difference.

One by one if we shine our lights with positive energy we can illuminate the entire world.

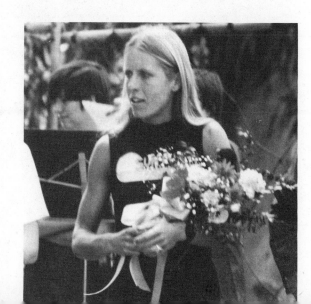

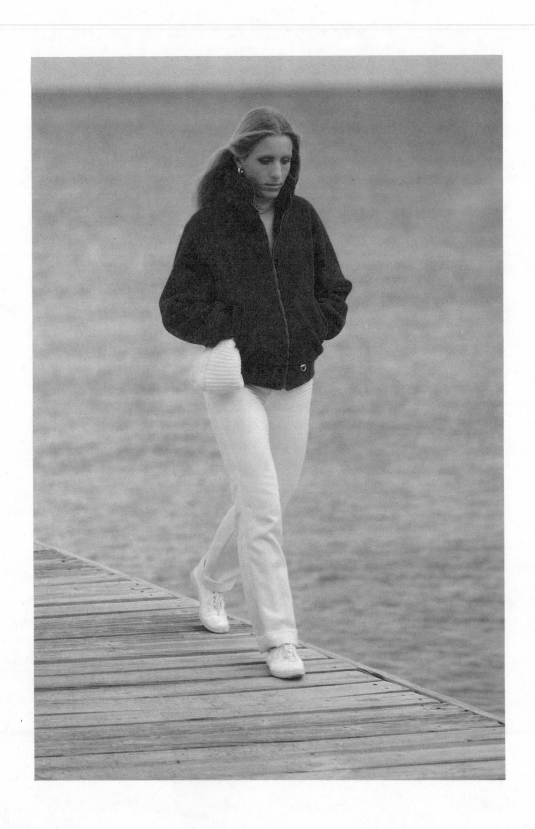

Epilogue

Strong women are not new to the world. In Greek mythology, Hippomenes had to chase the goddess Atalanta in a race to the wire.

More recently—a scant few hundred years ago—our foremothers landed on the east coast of North America and, with our equally strong forefathers, trudged over to the west coast because they heard California might be a nice place to live.

And these women were not sitting in the oxcart, filing their nails, during the trek. In most cases they were trudging alongside the oxcart, possibly carrying the family's china cabinet while they were at it.

Science and technology have surely conquered the geographical frontiers of our globe. Men and women make jokes in outer space for national TV, and you can melt snow in a microwave oven at the South Pole. So we're finding out that perhaps the last conquerable frontiers are our own personal, inner, and physical selves.

In such times of increasing mechanization, population, and military escalation, it becomes even more important to exercise control over some aspects of life in general. You may not be able to change the whole world, but you can certainly change yourself.

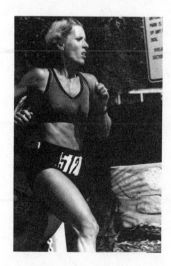

People who don't exercise never find their full potential. Exercising your body is like paying rent. Sure, there are other things you'd probably rather spend your money on first. But if you don't take care of it, sooner or later you don't have anywhere left to live.

Times are changing for the better, though. Just look at where we've been. Take Hollywood, for instance. As a mirror of our culture, the movies have given us many images of self-perception.

In early Hollywood, there were "men's men." Men heroes who were big and strong; ex-Olympians like Johnny Weissmuller, a Tarzan who made men swell their heads in pride, and women swell their heads with fantasy.

Later male stars were not classic beauties facially—Charles Bronson and Clint Eastwood, for instance—but they had "rugged good looks." Even though their faces were craggy, they had great physiques and they were tough. The Mr. Average-Guy-in-the-Street could therefore pump out a few hundred push-ups and chin-ups in the basement and still attain flattering comparisons to the stars at the beach when July rolled around.

Not so with the female stars of the silver screen. Female movie stars of the past have been "men's women," and certainly not "women's women."

Let me explain. Women are men's women when they have curves in all the right places. They were born gorgeous and could look glamorous in their movie roles, lipstick intact, even if the script called for a flop in a mud puddle.

Marilyn Monroe was a good example. She was man's woman. She was voluptuous. She was undeniably sexy, and men adored her. Women agreed to like her, only because she drove their men crazy, and she had looks they would scratch her eyes out for.

But lets face it: the divine Marilyn was **never** a woman's woman. Unlike the male screen stars, to whom the average guy could relate with a few manly flexes in front of the bathroom mirror, the female screen stars provided nothing the average woman could relate to. Honey, either you're born that way, or forget it!

At present, however, times are changing. Little girls and boys are now seeing Mommy doing sit-ups on the living room floor each morning. Role models are emerging—role models of women as something quite different from the bazooka buxomness of yesteryear's Hollywood pinup.

Into the eighties and nineties, we are seeing women's women in fashion, film, and finance. They stride confidently through the pages of slick magazines. They dress and shape their bodies to fit their new ideal of feminine beauty: strength.

108

Still, we have yet to see a megastar female who totally represents the new feminine ideal the way past screen stars embodied the fleshy role.

At this point, the marketplace is rampant with former sex symbols jumping on the fitness bandwagon and finding the diversion a lucrative pastime.

But it's only a matter of time before the camera pans to the front of the bandwagon and captures the starlets-to-be, who have been pulling the bandwagon all along. Real women, who are as tough as they are sexy.

Certainly there is now a women's athletic movement, and women historically have never done things in groups. Men have charged off together by the thousands in crusades throughout time. There has always been "boys' night out." The original Greek Olympic games were for men only. (Women caught viewing the spectacle were executed.)

Yet one year, standing at a starting line in Central Park, there were six thousand women behind me in line to run a 6.2 mile road race. We're talking about thousands of women all agreeing to do the same thing at the same time. That in itself has got to be history in the making.

One of the basic ideas behind women's lib was to achieve socioeconomic freedom for women, and freedom from male domination.

However, the danger in that situation was that there was often a transference, rather than a removal, of slavedom. Women soon became slaves to the movement, and still suffered because of the lack of personal freedom.

Women were still vulnerable as a group, and this traditional vulnerability stemmed from the lack of female physicalness. Sure, you can campaign for equal rights and open your own doors, and phone your own dates. But when you have to wait for your man to come home to open your own pickle jar because you're too weak to do it yourself, there's definitely something missing.

Lets face it: it's the little things in life that count. And all the little things add up to big things.

Change starts on the inside, and then works toward the outside. The athletic movement has taught women by the millions that physical strength allows for inner peace and happiness. Men and women run and lift weights and sweat together, and have discovered that fitness knows no gender. The reality of an honest working of muscles has caused an equality born of self-respect and the mutuality of the experience.

Of course, other factors in our social evolution cannot be ignored. Some may say that it wasn't suffragism, or even the women's athletic movement, as much as the impetus from science that changed us.

In the sixties, with women finally freed from the biological imperative via the pill, female socioeconomic freedom was exponentially multiplied. However, as our historical perspective is augmented by time, there will be even more answers, and perhaps even more questions.

Even so, with this new total package, complete with better jobs, more independence, muscle fatigue, and a training heart rate, women are realizing that beauty is indeed heaven-sent, but can be earth-improved. With sweat. Regardless of what Hollywood or anyone else has to say about it.

The ideal of the athletic body beautiful, nurtured so long ago in the myths of an ancient civilization, is here again—this time as part of our birthright.

Strong women are not new to this world; yet with the pursuit of strength as part of our birthright—male or female—new and exciting challenges remain for us.

My hope is that our seeking hearts will always find the true gentleness that comes from strength.

And wishing you the beauty of that strength always.

Sincerely,

GAYLE OLINEKOVA

It is not the critic who counts, not the man who points out how the strong man stumbled, or where the doer of deeds could have done them better.

The credit belongs to the man who is actually in the arena; whose face is marred by dust and sweat and blood; who strives valiantly; who errs and comes short again and again; who knows the great enthusiasms, the great devotions, and spends himself in a worthy cause; who, at the best, knows in the end the triumph of high achievement; and who, at the worst, at least fails while daring greatly, so that his place shall never be with those cold and timid souls who know neither victory nor defeat.

—Theodore Roosevelt

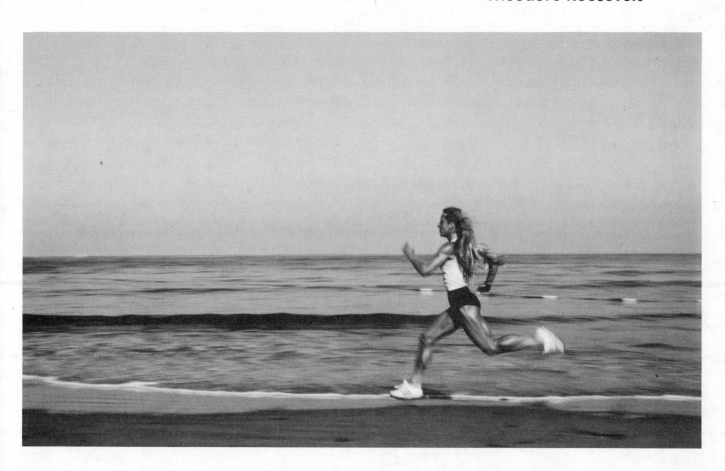